AF255726

Jumping to the Skies

Jumping to the Skies

Additional Lessons from Parkinson's Disease

ALLAN HUGH COLE JR.

CASCADE *Books* · Eugene, Oregon

JUMPING TO THE SKIES
Additional Lessons from Parkinson's Disease

Cascade Books
An Imprint of Wipf and Stock Publishers
199 W. 8th Ave., Suite 3
Eugene, OR 97401

www.wipfandstock.com

PAPERBACK ISBN: 978-1-6667-4818-5
HARDCOVER ISBN: 978-1-6667-4819-2
EBOOK ISBN: 978-1-6667-4820-8

Cataloguing-in-Publication data:

Names: Cole, Allan Hugh, Jr., author; foreword by Davis Phinney.

Title: Jumping to the skies : additional lessons from Parkinson's Disease / Allan Hugh Cole, Jr.

Description: Eugene, OR: Cascade Books, 2023 | Includes bibliographical references.

Identifiers: ISBN 978-1-6667-4818-5 (paperback) | ISBN 978-1-6667-4819-2 (hardcover) | ISBN 978-1-6667-4820-8 (ebook)

Subjects: LCSH: Parkinson's disease—Patients—Biography. | Parkinson's disease—Patients—Rehabilitation.

Classification: RC382 .C7726 2023 (print) | RC382 (ebook)

MAY 17, 2023 11:48 AM

For the late Michael Adams, Jim Davis, Dean Engelage,
Tom Goodrum, Mat Hamlin, Ethan Henderson, Dan Roberts,
Jordan Steiker, and Dan Stultz

"There are two kinds of teachers: the kind that fill you with so much quail shot that you can't move, and the kind that just gives you a little prod behind and you jump to the skies."

—ROBERT FROST

"Wherever you are, it is your friends who make your world."

—WILLIAM JAMES

Contents

Preface

If a prolonged illness changes your life, an incurable illness transforms it. My transformation began in the fall of 2016, at the age of forty-eight, with a diagnosis of young-onset Parkinson's disease. Progressive, degenerative, and currently incurable, over the course of many years Parkinson's can rob your body of movement and of many other physical, emotional, and mental functions that most of us take for granted.

My knowledge of illness has also changed. Intellectual knowledge, cultivated through years of study in philosophy, theology, psychology, and social work, has turned personal and led to existential understanding. I have gone from knowing a great deal about illness to understanding it subjectively and experientially, from the inside; the point being that one may *know* a lot, for a long time, while *understanding* comparatively little. I have come to rely more and more on what I understand, or seek to understand, to help me make meaning of a life with Parkinson's disease.

As was the case with my previous book, *Discerning the Way: Lessons from Parkinson's Disease* (Cascade, 2021), the chapters in this book began with posts on my blog, PD Wise (pdwise.com), and the chapters move back and forth in time and need not be read in any particular order.

As illness transforms us it can also teach us. Parkinson's has taught me the difference between living and being alive. The latter requires hearing the tick of your life's clock and learning to welcome it because it prompts savoring and utilizing each second you have.

Acknowledgments

If adding to *what* I understand about life with Parkinson's boosts me, relying more on *who* I know sustains me.

Rodney Clapp, my wise and perceptive editor at Cascade and a friend for many years, gifted me his guidance and wisdom and thus helped this become a better book. Indeed, the entire team at Cascade enriched this project, as they always do, especially Matt Wimer, managing editor, Jonathan Hill, typesetter, and Shannon Carter, cover designer. I remain grateful to work with them.

Elizabeth Gaucher, principal at Longridge Editors and a dear friend since our days at Davidson College, read many of the essays in this book, provided keen insights, and, as she has for years, helped me understand more and write better.

My friend, the late Michael Adams, read much of what I wrote about Parkinson's disease and he observed on multiple occasions that my family and friends are my primary muses. As one who also lived with Parkinson's, Michael helped me be a better writer and person.

Two of my colleagues in the Steve Hicks School of Social Work (SHS) at The University of Texas at Austin, namely, Mia Vinton, my executive assistant, and Stacey Jordan, my chief of staff, help me manage the rhythms and demands of my professional life and, among many other contributions, help me find time to write. I am grateful to work with both of them, and with the entire faculty and staff of the SHS.

Acknowledgments

My wife, Tracey, our daughters, Meredith and Holly, as well as my parents, Allan and Jeri Cole, with love and grace, keep adjusting to new ways of enjoying life, thinking about the future, and, importantly, living in the moment, all of which have been spawned by Parkinson's disease. Individually and collectively, they help me ensure that Parkinson's disruptions never carry the day while bringing the greatest joy and meaning to my life.

The philosopher William James, perhaps best known for his devotion to a philosophy of pragmatism and one of my intellectual heroes, taught me that "Wherever you are, it is your friends who make your world." Along with my family, among the many friends who have helped make my world with Parkinson's, and who help sustain me in it, are Jim Davis, Dean Engelage, Tom Goodrum, Mat Hamlin, Ethan Henderson, Dan Roberts, Jordan Steiker, and Dan Stultz.

Jim and I work together and share an appreciation for The University of Texas at Austin, the writings of Ralph Waldo Emerson, and the reflective life. Dean is my go-to for many things, especially those related to leadership. Tom has been my friend since our days at Davidson College, and he's one of the first people I told that I have Parkinson's. Mat and Dan (Roberts), both valued friends, share my love of boating and other outdoor activities, and our families have grown up together. I met Ethan in March of 2018, at an event hosted by the Michael J. Fox Foundation for Parkinson's Research, and as one who also lives with young-onset Parkinson's, he's been my closest comrade when navigating our respective paths with this illness. Jordan and I met many years ago when I invited him to give a talk about his work as a law school professor and to share his expertise in constitutional law. Since then, we have been close companions, confidantes, and reliable friends through joyous and heartbreaking experiences. Dan (Stultz) and I share a diagnosis of Parkinson's, a love of Texas, and a friendship that brings me great joy, meaning, and hope. As Shakespeare observed, "Words are easy, like the wind; faithful friends are hard to find."

An Anniversary Letter to My Daughters

October 26, 2020

Dear Holly and Meredith,

It's difficult to believe it has been four years since my Parkinson's diagnosis. I have never been one to make a big fuss over anniversaries, just ask Mom. But it feels important to write you this letter and share some things I have on my mind. Things I have realized in the last four years.

The first year with Parkinson's was the most difficult one because, as you know, I did not tell anyone I have this illness, including Grams and Papa, and both of you. I learned a lot in that year, including that it isn't good to hold our pain inside or to hide our feelings from those we love most. Honestly, being secretive about my Parkinson's took more of a toll on me than Parkinson's did. In hindsight, I wish I had been ready to share what I was going through sooner; it took me some time to understand the importance of not going through this alone.

I have challenging moments; you probably see some of them. But so many more moments are full of gratitude, happiness, and hope. I hope you see those, too.

You know I finally gave up my dream to pitch in the major leagues, preferably for the Astros, but, thankfully, my physical challenges remain manageable. Some things *are* harder to do, such as buttoning a shirtsleeve (you know this because you help me sometimes), getting a good night's sleep, and keeping my symptoms at bay when I'm under stress, but I can still do what I have always done and I hope this continues for many more years. My doctors tell me it should.

I don't know what future days will entail, of course, but that would be true if I didn't have Parkinson's, too; and it's that way for everyone, really.

I do know that we have generous and supportive people in our lives, which helps a lot: our family and friends, my colleagues and doctors, and especially others who live with Parkinson's. Together they help me find ways to push through the more challenging moments, keep me moving forward, and focus on living the one and only life any of us have.

You help me too, you know, just by sharing your awesomeness. Just by being you.

You know I love to write, and that I write a lot these days about my life with Parkinson's. Writing about Parkinson's helps me find meaning and purpose in having it, and also helps me heal and live better. I also write about my experiences because I want to help others discover their own meaning, purpose, and healing, whether they live with Parkinson's or face other challenges or uncertainties.

You also know I love to teach. As a teacher, I tend to look for the *lessons* I am learning from Parkinson's. So far, these have been lessons on trust, patience, discipline, authenticity, vulnerability, values, injustice, kindness, compassion, gratitude, hope, and so much more.

As is true for you in school, I do not have all of these lessons down pat or learned once and for all. And I cannot learn them by cramming, copying others, or by trying to memorize them, either. Instead, these lessons unfold each day, little by little—through living life, facing its setbacks, recognizing its beauty, and nurturing ourselves and others through love.

That's one of the biggest lessons so far.

I think you'll agree that with a slow unfolding of these lessons comes more understanding, but sometimes more confusion, too. Learning often happens this way. Like with your Spanish or math! Right?

I am learning each day as I go, gradually becoming better at understanding Parkinson's and better at living with it, too, even as new questions come up, confuse me, and require me to keep exploring for answers.

There are always new lessons to learn.

You were young when Parkinson's rudely joined our family, and now you are older, thirteen and almost fifteen. Wow, what a quick four years.

I don't want to make a big fuss over this anniversary. But I do want you to know that you provide me precious daily gifts of love and hope, joy and fun, gratitude and expectation—and all of this began the moment I knew you were coming into the world. Together, you fill my heart and soul.

Especially when you laugh at my dad jokes.

No doubt, you will face difficulties in life. Everyone does. Mom and I wish we could prevent these difficulties and spare you the pain they bring, but no parent can do that. No life has only the easy stuff to deal with.

Just remember that you do not have to face the difficulties alone, or hide your feelings, or carry your pain inside.

Ever.

Remember this, too. The dad who tells corny jokes and loves you so much also learns, grows, lives a good life, feels joy, and finds peace in the face of his own challenges; and from personal hardships, whether our own or others', we can learn some of life's most important lessons.

So, who is watching the World Series with me?

It's our anniversary!

Love,

Dad

···   2   ···

Ungated

Isolation

THE RUSTED CHAIN LINK fence sags in multiple places while its tall
iron gate clanks in the Texas wind. Weathered metal letters above
the gate spell out "A. S. H. Cemetery."

This gate provides entry to the Austin State Hospital Cemetery, an eleven-acre, minimally maintained field surrounded by
urban life in central Austin. Despite being in use for longer than a
century and having more than three thousand people buried there,
few gravestones dot this mostly barren and unexceptional terrain.
Instead, the graves are marked with small, numbered, concrete
slabs, meager reminders of seemingly unexceptional lives.

Loneliness

A gated community of forgotten souls symbolizes the isolation
and loneliness that many people experience, and not only those
who lived with mental illness, who died at the Austin State Hospital, and whose remains were unclaimed. Theirs might be the more
severe experiences, but they are surely not the only ones. In fact,
as Dorothy Day put it, "We have all known the long loneliness."[1]

1. Day, *Long Loneliness*, 286.

Indeed, we have. Did you know that more than one-third of adults aged forty-five and older feel lonely and that nearly one in four adults aged sixty-five and older are socially isolated?[2] Social isolation means a lack of contact with other persons and an absence of companionship and support.

Loneliness means feeling like an outsider, as though one does not belong, or lacking in desired intimacy, such as friendship, companionship, or romance.[3] Note that these figures predate the current global pandemic, where COVID-19 and loneliness go together like rusted fences and forgotten souls.

We also know that loneliness as well as social isolation puts people at risk for serious medical conditions, especially those over age fifty. We know, too, that those who live with Parkinson's not only experience social isolation and loneliness (about half of us do, in fact), but that those who *are* lonely tend to have a more severe course of disease progression.[4]

So why are we lonely?

The reasons for isolation vary, but among those with Parkinson's, they include things such as a lack of confidence or sense of significance; self-consciousness about a loss of functioning or changed appearance; and underestimating or devaluing what one has left to contribute to one's work, social networks, or others' lives. The studies consistently bear this out, as do my own experiences and those of my friends.

For example, my heart ached when I once heard a close friend with Parkinson's who struggled with dyskinesia say, "Why would I attend that party? I'll just embarrass myself and make everyone there feel uncomfortable?"[5]

2. National Academies of Sciences, Engineering, and Medicine, *Social Isolation and Loneliness in Older Adults.*

3. Cornwell and Waite, "Social Disconnectedness, Perceived Isolation, and Health among Older Adults."

4. Rukovets, "It's a Triple Threat."

5. Dyskinesia refers to involuntary movements of the arms, legs, trunk, or face, and includes erratic rocking, jerking, swaying, or fidgeting. Dyskinesia is a side effect of Parkinson's medications, and not a symptom of the disease itself.

When we feel this way about ourselves, we can begin constructing barriers to relationships and connections that we need most, not only to sustain our health but to give us life. Building these fences and gates around us, though seemingly self-protective and surely an understandable response, actually robs us of much more than Parkinson's ever should.

I know this because I have felt like my friend did, and my inclination, like his, was to stay away from the party.

But it turns out that we get invited to only so many parties, and that we do not enjoy unlimited opportunities for human connection, relationship, and love. Why? Because we all get only one life to live.

Connections

Picturing that rusted fence and clanking gate, I got myself dressed, called my friend, and my wife Tracey and I picked him up and carried him (almost literally) to that party. He had some dyskinetic wiggles. I was stiff, fatigued from a lack of sleep, and not bringing my A game, either. Still, with our limitations, imperfections, and insecurities tethered to Parkinson's disease, we got ourselves to the party, stood among other limited, imperfect, and insecure people, some of whom were surely lonely, and we enjoyed good food and drink, even better conversation, and lived our life.

Our life.

The *only* life we get.

Maybe one day I will share this experience with the souls in that cemetery.

To let them know they are remembered.

3

Making It

Speaking

ONE SATURDAY MORNING I wait in line at my local bakery, ready to pick up cinnamon rolls for my family. I'm standing the obligatory six feet behind a young boy and his father, the smells of coffee and fresh baked goods wafting through the air. Neither the loss of an ability to smell that comes with Parkinson's nor a COVID-19-mandated mask can fully stop the warm sugar, spices, and yeast from reaching my brain.

The excited dark-haired boy wears a red soccer jersey, and from the back of it I learn his name: Cooper. A freshly scraped knee tells part of his story, as does his energy and attempts to push through several starts and stops in his speech.

Cooper stutters.

Recounting a pre-pandemic soccer game for his father and maybe for me, too, he speaks especially of how he helped his team win on a penalty kick. Cooper's voice gets louder as he acts out the scene.

"It was awe–, awe–, awesome, Dad," he says, before describing, first, how he took notice of the goalkeeper's position in front of the goal, and then, how he thought he could get the soccer ball past him, and *then* how nervous he was when lining up to take the kick. Though his speech challenges ebb and flow as he speaks, they never get in the way of his infectious excitement.

"And . . . and . . . and . . . and I knew it was good the moment it left my foot, Dad. I *knew* it."

His attentive father nods along. "I had no doubt you'd make it, Coop," he says, "no doubt at all." Then he extends both arms toward his son and waits for a double fist bump. A father's smiling eyes rest above a dark blue COVID mask.

Reflecting

I have thought a lot about Cooper and his father since this Saturday morning encounter. Perhaps it is because I know that some people who stutter have a dopamine problem, just as everyone with Parkinson's does. With Parkinson's you have too little dopamine in your brain, while some who stutter have too much.

Maybe I keep thinking about Cooper because many of us with Parkinson's eventually face our own speech problems—challenges that we have to integrate into our relationships and lives if we cannot push past them. I have in mind the challenges of speaking too rapidly, too softly, or with hoarseness, slurring words as well as stuttering. All of this, and more, can happen with Parkinson's.

Resolving

Mainly, though, Cooper's courage and resolve draw me to him, just as his father's obvious love and devotion do. Despite a joyous view of soccer and, in the main, I gather, of life, I suppose Cooper has also experienced the hurt of teasing and frustration over not being able to communicate as efficiently as he would like; and I wonder if someday he will fear not gaining more control over his stutter.

Here, especially, is where familial love, as well as the encouragement of others, weighs in and fosters courage for pushing through the challenges—courage that, otherwise, we might not know we have.

Courage and resolve. Love and devotion. A boy who stutters, his faithful father, and a bystander with Parkinson's disease; all of us with smiling eyes, six feet apart but with fewer than six degrees of neurologic separation between us.

Like his father, I believe Cooper will make it.

I believe I will, too.

4

Being Happy

Being Happy

Parkinson's brings surprises. Some unexpected events are pleasant, such as meeting extraordinary folks who live with this illness, while other unexpected events are unpleasant, such as the various symptoms that come with losing dopamine in your brain. It's a mixed bag. Still, when people ask how I'm doing, I often quip, "For a fifty-two-year-old man with a progressive and incurable neurologic condition, I'm doing just fine."

And I mean it.

This brings me to one of the biggest surprises about having Parkinson's disease (PD): Most of the people I know who live with it are happy. They're not happy they have Parkinson's—it sucks big time, for all of us—but happy in the ways we think of anyone being happy, namely, living satisfied, contented, with purpose, and experiencing joy, even as their struggles with this illness remain challenging and real.

Recently I heard an acquaintance say, "It comes down to my realization that I just want to be happy; that this is what life's all about." He made this remark as a group of us met on Zoom and discussed the pandemic.

He is not alone in his perspective; I suppose most people would identify happiness as a chief end in life. We want to be happy, just as we want happiness for our children, other loved ones, our friends, and, on our better days, even for those who have angered or hurt us. We recognize happiness as a basic good, for everyone, and that pursuing happiness remains part and parcel of being human. Still, *how* we pursue happiness and *where* we look for it can differ, whether living with illness or not.

Misassumptions

Many people assume that those of us living with a chronic illness must not be happy. How could we be, the thinking goes, given the ongoing challenges of managing life when feeling poorly? It's a fair question, but it's misguided.

British philosopher Havi Carel, who lives with a chronic lung condition, challenges what lies behind this assumption, namely, that a good life requires good health, and she pushes back on those who would view illness as a disaster that strikes and essentially ruins one's life.[1]

She tells the story of getting into a taxi late one night after a full day of work at an academic conference. Because of her chronic lung condition, she carried a cylinder of oxygen with her. As the oxygen passed through tubes and into her nose, its distinct sounds filled the quiet cab, and after driving a short distance, the taxi driver inquired about the apparatus. When Carel explained what it was and that it helped her breathe with a chronic lung condition, the cab driver's response was, "I pity you." As she departed the car, he promised to pray for her.

Though many of us welcome prayers, I have yet to meet anyone with Parkinson's who wants pity. This is because those who live with PD often tell a different story than the taxi driver assumed about illness. In fact, research shows that both disabled and chronically ill people seem to have only somewhat lower levels of well-being (which includes happiness) compared to healthy people, while many studies find no difference in levels of reported

---

1. Carel, *Phenomenology of Illness*, 131.

well-being between groups of people with a variety of medical conditions and healthy controls.[2]

Other studies demonstrate, more or less, what health economists and happiness researchers have found occurs, namely, that after a year or so of living with a chronic illness, unless it results in a severe disturbance in the way one lives, one should expect to live as happily as one did prior to becoming ill.[3] However, what becomes the *basis* for happiness certainly can change.

Importantly, life with an illness is not *necessarily* a happy life, but it *may* be a happy life if one develops certain perspectives on illness and embraces particular ways of living with it. Similarly, healthy people may live exceedingly *unhappy* lives.[4] Also, although illness remains unwelcome for all of us, in our fears about becoming ill we neglect to consider the opportunities it presents for learning to live well *because* of illness, which includes being happy.

Rethinking Happiness

Is happiness, then, really our chief end in life; or could it be something else?

Leo Rosten, a twentieth-century screenwriter and humorist thought so, noting, "The purpose of life is *not* to be happy. It is to be useful, to be honorable, to be compassionate, to have it make some difference that you have lived and lived well."[5]

My experience has been that living with Parkinson's, and maybe any chronic illness, has most to do with discovering one's usefulness going forward—for living, working, learning, relating, whatever we deem important—but especially with finding compassion, for others as well as ourselves.

This brings me to my friend and colleague, Andrea. A person of relatively few words, she listens as well as anyone I have met, and

2. Carel, *Phenomenology of Illness*, 134.

3. Carel, *Phenomenology of Illness*, 135.

4. Carel, *Phenomenology of Illness*, 132.

5. Rosten, *Words to Live By*, 2.

she also has a rare ability for discernment matched by an enviable dry sense of humor. The world needs more of both. You sense in Andrea a grounded spirit, confident resolve, and principled kindness that make those around her kinder and more discerning.

Last week, she informed me, in a rather matter-of-fact way, that she would need to take some additional time off from work over the holidays, between the fall and spring semesters, because she will be recovering from surgery after donating a kidney to her friend.

Andrea does not live with Parkinson's. But if she did, I think she would be happy. I believe she would continue to have experiences of deep satisfaction and contentment, which are more lasting and firmly established than what we might typically think informs happiness, and I am confident that she would look at illness as something that brings opportunities for meaning, growth, compassion, joy—happiness, along with many, many surprises.

I also think she would point to Leo Rosten, noting that what he said is true, "The purpose of life is *not* to be happy. It is to be useful, to be honorable, to be compassionate, to have it make some difference that you have lived and lived well."

5

Spiritual Questions

The Assignment

THE CLASS BEGINS AS many do these days, with young faces popping up on the computer screen. Everyone is muted and it's quiet, as though we have met on the moon. David, my close friend and colleague of fifteen years, has invited me to speak with college students taking a seminar he calls "Building a Happy Life." He has asked me to talk about my experience of living with Parkinson's, as a way of helping students think about how illness and happiness are not mutually exclusive, and especially about my spiritual path. David recognizes that, for many people, experiences of happiness and contentment remain tethered to their spiritual passions and commitments; and he wants students to have a conversation about this relationship.

The Background

I suppose my background is what led David to tap me for this assignment. Before becoming a professor in social work education, I taught for eleven years in a seminary, and before that, I served as a minister in three different congregations. Moreover, much of my research and writing relates to the intersections of philosophical and theological questions and concerns, on the one hand, and psychological or clinical questions and concerns on the other.

David introduces me to the class, and I share my story of being diagnosed four years earlier with young-onset Parkinson's, at the age of forty-eight. I speak about the actual diagnosis and of an initial misdiagnosis, of remaining silent for nearly a year, of the pain that came with trying in secrecy to adjust to a new life, of fear and anxiety about the future—all of that. I also speak about how eventually I began not only to cope with this illness but to make it part of a rich, meaningful, and happy life.

The Questions

It's clear that only a couple of the students have personal experience with Parkinson's, but many of them can relate my experience to others' experiences of illness—whether belonging to a family member, friend, or themselves.

After I speak for a few minutes, the students begin asking questions, about Parkinson's, my experience, and how it has affected my spiritual path. Three questions garner particular interest on the part of several of the students: *Were you angry? Did you ever ask "Why me?" Did you ever question your beliefs?*

A Response

On the first question, I tell them I was profoundly sad to learn I have Parkinson's, but not angry. Honest. Anger, I say, links to feeling wronged or violated in some fashion, mistreated or hurt by someone, or to see any of these affecting another person whom we hold dear. Any of that is certainly grounds for anger.

But I experienced none of this. Just the opposite has been true.

Before Parkinson's and since, I have enjoyed good fortune and privilege in my life, as well as having supportive parents, a loving partner and children, compassionate friends, and generous colleagues.

Also, I get to make a living as I teach, learn from, and grow and serve with extraordinary people, every day I go to work—work, incidentally, that I would gladly do for free if I had other means by which to live and provide for my family.

I have also met hundreds of inspiring, decent, compassionate, and dedicated people who live with Parkinson's, as well as those who support and care for them. Not only this, but I now experience a richness of humanity and a joy for living that, frankly, I never knew was possible before Parkinson's knocked.

It's hard to feel angry when considering any of this.

Am I sad? Of course! And occasionally, still brokenhearted. But not angry. As my wife and children will confirm, I frequently cite Mark Twain's observation about anger. It is "an acid that can do more harm to the vessel in which it is stored than to anything on which it is poured."

I'm not suggesting that one should never be angry over an illness. Anger is a core human emotion, and we must learn to feel it and express it if we are to let go of it, or, at least, not allow it to harm us. Even so, learning to distinguish between my own sadness and anger has been a great gift. When I'm angry, it's often the case that I need to turn my anger into sadness, to grieve, and then move forward.

Another Response

Concerning the second question, asking *Why me?* is surely understandable when facing illness or other hardships. There have been times in my life when I asked the question myself. However, I do not recall ever asking this question as it relates to my having Parkinson's. I have discovered that whenever it's asked, *Why me?* is rarely about a search for a definitive answer, and more often a cry of pain, a lament over one's experience or situation, an expression of feeling helpless and vulnerable—all of which are fundamentally human.

Illness can visit anyone, at any time; and eventually, it touches everyone. I became more fully aware of this fact of life as a young minister, standing at bedsides and gravesides, and long before I got Parkinson's disease. Sadly, illness is simply a part of human existence. It's also a part of life that can easily be overlooked or even denied as long as we and those we love can breeze through our days with good health. But recognizing illness as a fact of life is different than thinking it singles out certain people, or it's part of a divine plan or one's destiny or anything like that.

I don't know why people get sick when they do. In most cases, it probably relates to genes, environment, and behavior. I do know that while being ill is never intrinsically good, many good things can come about as a result of living with illness.

Like the time I spent with David's class.

As this class period draws to a close, I am grateful to have the opportunity to think with young, bright minds about these important life questions.

And Another

After class, I realize I didn't answer the question about how my illness has touched my spiritual beliefs as thoroughly as I wanted to.

I wish I had put it this way.

That we live in sacred, even holy, spaces touched by divine goodness and love, has never felt truer to me. Neither has my awareness ever been keener that this goodness and love endure, especially in the darkest and most painful moments of life.

I have spent decades of my life searching for answers to the students' questions—which have been my questions, too, and still are sometimes. I have spent equal time hoping for glimpses of the divine. The more salient answers and spottings have come with embracing and even appreciating the ambiguity of illness, with accepting the messiness of *Why?* and, most importantly, in seeking to live in fierce solidarity with others whose lives are touched by illness, loss, or pain, whatever the reasons or causes.

A few days later, still reflecting on this meaningful experience offered by my kind friend David and his bright and thoughtful students, I wrote a poem I call "Faith," and it includes these lines:

> *. . . Some years later came infirmity's call.*
> *In losses and crosses, there I saw*
> *That stated beliefs never satisfy me,*
> *But actions and love help eyes to see*
> *The sacred is true, for others, for me.*
> *. . . With keener vision, now I see:*
> *Faith equals what the prophet decreed,*
> *Loving justice, kindness, humility—these three.*
> *In this way, the sacred endures for me.*[1]

My parting words to David's students are that I suppose a happy life is one with space for health *and* illness, joy *and* sorrow, answers *and* questions, and really that any life needs all of these if it's to be real, not to mention faithful.

---

1. This poem includes an allusion to Micah 6:8, *The Holy Bible* (New Revised Standard Version).

Memories and Realities

A Boy

It's 1977 and I'm nine years old. The intense North Texas sun shines hard on my dirty, sweat-coated face as I ride through a steep berm at Rabbit Run Motocross Park. My coveted yellow and black Yamaha YZ80 spits out dark, loamy dirt from its back tire as I straighten my handlebars and meet a long straightaway heading toward a series of tall jumps.

My faithful dad stands just outside the track behind the bright orange plastic fencing and strings of multicolored pennant flags that mark its boundaries. A frequent presence when I ride, he gives me two thumbs up as I pull back hard on the throttle, preparing to soar over those jumps and make another lap around the track.

I can ride like this for hours and I often do.

A Man

Forty-three years later, I head north on Congress Avenue in Austin with the Texas Capitol lying straight ahead. It's early on a Saturday morning with hardly a car on the road, and now I'm riding a different motorcycle, a beautiful red Suzuki I have just purchased, and I feel like I did at nine years old.

It's been more than a decade since I got the motorcycle bug again. After years of lobbying my wife, Tracey, and after taking a motorcycle safety course, buying a top-rated helmet, and agreeing to a list of rules as long as my arm, she has finally given me her consent. It's far from an enthusiastic endorsement, mind you, but it's heartfelt, kind, generous, and the green light I have sought for years.

We both know the reasons I should not be riding a motorcycle. At the same time, we know that everyone needs to attend to certain things if they are to live, assessing risks and rewards that come with them, yes, but never diminishing what offers joy, freedom, and a sense of being fully alive.

There's also something about having a progressive and incurable illness that gets your attention, that confronts you with an acute awareness of life's ticking clock, of how little you are guaranteed while on this clock, and of what's at stake when you opt to live as more of a spectator of what you love than a participant in it.

A Decision

Admittedly, I did not tell many people I bought a motorcycle. I feared their judgment, or that they would assume I had lost my mind. A few of those I told or who saw me riding around our neighborhood likely wondered if I was having the proverbial midlife crisis. You know, an aha moment or series of moments that some folks in middle age experience when they realize they do not have unlimited time on this earth.

But these critical turning points, these crises, can motivate us, whether constructively or otherwise, to stake new claims on life, to experience certain things while we still can, and to embrace a line in a well-known movie, "We either get busy living or get busy dying."[1]

To whatever extent I have stood in judgment of others and their personal choices—such as a fifty-something buying a

1. See Darabont, dir., *Shawshank Redemption*.

motorcycle or a convertible sports car—I do so less often since learning I have Parkinson's disease.

This brings me to share a decision I made a few weeks after buying the motorcycle. I decided to sell it to someone who feels as delighted to get it as I did. There are several reasons for my decision and I won't rehearse them all. Simply put, I'm a fifty-two-year-old man living with Parkinson's disease, and while I can still ride just fine, I cannot ride at Rabbit Run.

A Gift

Willa Cather wrote, "Some memories are realities and are better than anything that can ever happen to one again."[2] I had experiences and created memories on that red Suzuki that will stay with me, just like the memories of joy and freedom—of love—I had as a young boy riding with my dad. Parkinson's will never touch any of this.

Never.

Of course, some of the more meaningful and rewarding experiences in life come with risk. Whether riding a motorcycle, starting a new job, entering into a romantic relationship, or giving birth to a child, no meaningful life can be risk-free. No abundant life remains entirely safe.

Still, we all have to make choices about what risks we can tolerate. We choose the risks worth taking, those we do best to forego, and those we can leave to others and then live vicariously through them. It can take some time to make these kinds of choices. Sometimes, it can take forty-three years or longer.

That Tracey consented to my getting the Suzuki is something that only deepens my love for her. As she has for over thirty years, she looked into my eyes and understood.

I doubt I'll ever need to ask for her consent to ride again, but I'm keeping my helmet, just in case.

I'm also lobbying her for a convertible.

2. Cather, *My Ántonia*, 216.

Staring into the Fire

Snow Days

IT's JUST BEFORE 4 PM on a cold, wintry day in Austin, and a few patches of heavy wet snow still sit on the St. Augustine grass in my front yard. The previous day's rare snowfall brought scores of neighbors outside and put joy on faces of all ages. It also caused widespread power outages across the city, leaving my family, and thousands of others, without any electricity or heat.

As the day's last light slips away, I break out flashlights and headlamps, battery-powered lanterns, and several candles, and my wife, Tracey, our two teenage daughters, and I prepare a simple dinner. Afterward, we all sit in front of our fireplace with its hissing gas logs and talk for what seems like longer than we have talked in a very long time.

No cell phones, laptops, or binge-watched TV shows. No FaceTime or Zoom with friends. Not even a good book distracts us. Instead, we sit close to each other by the fire, laughing and talking. We reminisce about the fun things we have done. We discuss issues of the day, our respective beliefs about things that matter to us, and a few other topics, too, all of which warm my soul and make me feel at home.

In moments like these, I forget I have Parkinson's.

Bridge Nights

After Tracey and the girls fall asleep wearing their winter coats and hats, I stay up and write for a bit, taking breaks to stare at the tall orange flames reaching for our chimney.

My mind drifts to Chris and Shae, a young couple we met just three weeks before. They looked to be in their late twenties, though it's hard to know for sure. Living in a tent and under an interstate bridge can age you quickly.

Tracey and I were delivering some food our girls had helped us prepare for people in situations like the one Chris and Shae faced. By this, I mean those living not far from where we live, but in what has become a community of survivors who spend their days and nights in tents and under plastic tarps tied between several shopping carts filled with all their possessions. "The homeless" remains a shorthand way of identifying this population, but "human beings who have no roof over their heads, who lack adequate food, and who live exposed not only to brutal weather but also to frequent threats of violence" is the more accurate and personal description.

We greeted Shae and Chris amid the loud hums of heavy traffic above us, various piles of discarded clothing and other debris, and a faint sour smell of urine. As we gave them bags of food and engaged in forced conversation, I noticed that Shae was pregnant, as did Tracey, who told them we would have more food in a couple of days. After another minute or two of awkward conversation and periods of silence, we wished them well, said goodbye, and returned home.

Fireside Thoughts

Nearly ten hours have passed since we lost power. It's almost midnight, and I can feel the temperature dropping as I stare into the fire. My eyes flit to Tracey and our girls bundled up in warm, clean clothes and covered by down sleeping bags, and I'm taken back to our encounter with Chris and Shae. Turning on my headlamp, I write this poem:

As heavy traffic drones above their heads,
A winter's sun begins to set,
Returning them to a nightly dread.
Their dirty tent under the interstate's bridge
Protects them some from wind and rain,
Though not from cold or fear, nor pain.
We speak of the child's pending birth, which
Puts a bent smile on her father's face
As we offer them food and I hope for grace.
Whispering to myself, "It should not be this way,"
I wonder if they will find a new place to stay,
Or have to settle for a bigger tent.

Future Memories

When I finish writing, I turn off my headlamp, close my battery-drained laptop, and again stare into the fire. My thoughts shift again.

It occurs to me that when I struggle with having Parkinson's and with how I can best live with it, or when I worry about what may lie ahead for my family and me, I want to remember the encounter with Shae and Chris. I want to remind myself of their burdens, their dearth of resources, their worries and fears; but also their courage and what may bring them happiness and hope. Also, I want to try my best to imagine what life is like for them day to day. I may not be able to imagine accurately, but I sure want to try.

I also want to remember them—Shae and Chris—in the hope that they and their newborn child are warm and safe, healthy and happy; and that they have begun to create new and better memories than those marking the day we met. I don't know their personal stories, and I wish I did. I know these stories include much more than living under a bridge. Or how they got there.

Which is not altogether different than the stories of those living with Parkinson's.

Most of all, I hope Shae and Chris are in a place that warms their souls and that they can call home.

Typos and 90-Degree Angles

Typos

IT'S LATE AND EVERYONE but me is fast asleep—my wife, Tracey, our girls, three dogs, and a bird. It's quiet, dark, and calm. A peaceful February cold surrounds our warm home. Having fallen asleep a couple of hours earlier, I am wide awake now and trying to make peace with an all too familiar experience that having Parkinson's provides.

Insomnia.

I decide I'll look through the page proofs for my new book, *Counseling Persons with Parkinson's Disease*, which will be released in just a few weeks. Each book I've written has a special place in my heart—after all, I write to know what I think—but none has been more meaningful than this book. From working with my editor and friend, Dana Bliss, to having my friend Elizabeth Gaucher and several close colleagues read the manuscript and give me feedback, to hoping it will help those who offer counsel to those of us living with an insidious disease—all of that makes this book particularly special and makes me eager to hold it in my hands.

Preparing to scroll through the pages, an incorrectly placed apostrophe catches my eye. In fact, atop the book's very first page, right there in front of God and everybody, it reads, *Counseling Person's with Parkinson's Disease.*

Person's!

I have a flashback to the third grade in Richardson, Texas, and to my teacher, Ms. Ora Lamb, whose expectations for proper spelling, not to mention grammar, have kept a hold on me for forty-five years.

For about forty-eight years, my age when diagnosed with Parkinson's, I would have lost even more sleep over this presumed error. I would have stewed over it and beat myself up for not catching it sooner, when there was still time to make changes. I'd probably also have had a few choice words to say about the copyeditor at my publisher, whose job it is to catch these errors and correct them before going to press. As Tracey pointed out three decades ago, not long after we met, "Allan likes things at 90-degree angles."

But that was before Parkinson's put lots of angles with differing degrees in my life. So, I calmly wrote an email to Fabian, the production manager at the publisher, told her what I had discovered, and asked if she could let me know whether someone had seen it and made the change before putting the book into production.

Then, I went to bed in hopes that I'd sleep through the night.

Imperfections

In my mid-twenties, the summer before my last year of seminary, I had the opportunity to take Hebrew at the Jewish Theological Seminary in New York. Those ten weeks remain some of the more interesting ones of my life, not because I became fluent in Hebrew (far from it), but because I learned so much about Judaism and its rich practices. One of them is the tradition when building a home of leaving a portion of it unfinished, a symbol of life's imperfections and unfinished state.[1] Years later, I'd learn of a similar tradition among the Navajo, who intentionally weave a "flaw" into their

---

1. https://templebethel.org/perfect-imperfections-by-rabbi-judith-schindler/.

rugs—a spirit-line, they call it—which reminds all who see it that life is never perfect.[2]

Parkinson's feels like living in this kind of unfinished state and having this type of flaw, both of which can serve to remind us that nothing is perfect—not health, nor relationships, nor jobs, nor plans we make, nor our possessions—nothing.

Life gets a lot easier and less stressful when we stop expecting otherwise. As Tolstoy put it, if you look for perfection, you'll never be content.

More Angles

When I check my email the next morning, Fabian has written me back. All is well. A final copyedit flagged the typo and corrected it. My title was as it should be.

Part of me wishes it had remained imperfect, just as I am, just as we all are. There is beauty to be found there, after all, and authenticity as well, both of which we see in unfinished homes or deliberately imperfect rugs that point us to what matters more in life than perfection: family, pets, friends, colleagues, meaningful work, books, those who live in solidarity when facing illness, and so much more.

Having Parkinson's has helped me see all of it more clearly.

The other part of me, the one schooled by Ms. Lamb and calmed by 90-degree angles, is glad the errant apostrophe was caught and removed. Dana will be, too, and so will Elizabeth.

After all, it was on the first page!

2. https://michellealexander.in/blogs/news/navajos.

Feeling at Home

Plans

FOR YEARS, I THOUGHT I would someday become an old-fashioned barber. I would have a little shop on Main Street in a sleepy community, maybe a college town. The shop would have one barber's chair, four or five chairs for those waiting, and several current newspapers and magazines for clients to read. I would offer haircuts and shaves at a reasonable price, only take walk-ins, and have free coffee and Cokes available to anyone who stopped by. My shop would be as much a hub for visiting with neighbors and talking about things that matter—such as politics, religion, books, and baseball—as a place to be coiffed. Most importantly, you could come as you are, with "bed head" or "hat head," and read the newspaper, sip coffee, visit with other customers, or even doze off if you felt the need.

Guides

His name was Mr. Kenneth Norton, and he wooed me to his craft in 1986. It was my first year of college in Davidson, North Carolina. As far as I know, Norton—that's what he asked us to call him—owned and operated the only barbershop in town, located directly across the street from the college. A local icon, Norton had cut the hair and shaved the faces of Davidson College students and other townsfolk for four decades, since 1942, and going to see him was both a step back in time and a rite of passage for many students. When I close my eyes, I can still smell Clubman aftershave colliding with baby powder, the result of Norton's soft boar's-hair brush touching the top of my ears and my neck, which stung after he shaved it with a straight razor. To borrow a term from the psychologist Erik H. Erikson, a visit to Norton's provided me with a sense of at-homeness in the world, of feeling significant and being cared for in the right place.

Norton was a masterful storyteller and he only knew how to cut hair one way. Short! I'm talking semi-buzz cuts in the era of big hair and mullets; we called it being "Nortonized." To step foot in his shop was to accept the fact that you would not need another haircut for quite some time; the only way to avoid this outcome was not letting him tell a long story, because he cut your hair until he finished telling the tale. If he had been a poet, think in terms of wanting to hear him recite a haiku as opposed to the *Iliad*.

Short hair notwithstanding, Norton made you look cool. But his vocation took hold of me because he seemed so content with what he did, so well-suited for his craft, and he earned a living making meaningful contributions to people's lives in a place that smelled good. Felt good. As an eighteen-year-old, I had no clue what I wanted to do with my life, but I had a sense of wanting a similarly satisfying path. I also decided that whatever I ended up doing, and however long I did it, retiring to the barbershop and "Allanizing" people should remain in my plans. As my wife, Tracey, will attest, for decades I spoke of this plan fairly often.

Home

But sometimes, plans change. Parkinson's hands and barbering are not a natural fit. Still, I enjoyed imagining the barber life for years and I admired those who claimed it for themselves.

Jayber Crow, novelist Wendell Berry's character who also happens to be a barber, says, "The music, while it lasted, brought a new world into being."[1] The music continues for me, with as much volume and tempo as ever, albeit in a different tune; and the world of the long-anticipated barbershop community has been replaced with the Parkinson's community and its world.

It turns out that they are not so different.

Both worlds offer opportunities for connection, friendship, laughter, telling stories, sharing burdens, and talking about things that matter. In both places, you can come as you are, stay for a while, and feel welcomed, valued, cared for, and even cool, regardless of how you look or move.

We do not know what will become of our plans or what worlds we will live in, and I find this true whether we are in our twenties, fifties, or beyond. Sometimes the unexpected worlds discovered turn out to be where we live more contented than we thought possible, surrounded by people and experiences that matter to us, and where, despite our lives and plans changing, we can feel at home.

1. Berry, *Jayber Crow*, 128.

Bittersweet Lane

Reflection

It's AFTER 7 AM when the new day's sunlight hits the shallow Frio River, which outlines a portion of Bittersweet Lane. This majestic place in the Texas Hill Country is owned by dear family friends, and they have invited my family and me to join them for a few days while our children are on Spring Break.

As I sit on the front porch of their small guest house with a warm cup of coffee in hand, the cool March breeze blows and wakes brushy hilltops lying a short distance across the river. A bird coos as the tranquil setting invites my reflection.

Pandemic

It's been exactly one year since COVID-19's destruction spread so quickly across the world; when life as we knew it abruptly changed. Seemingly overnight, human faces largely disappeared, as did human touch in the form of handshakes and hugs among colleagues and friends. For children and adults, friendships at once became more "socially distanced" and quickly morphed into smaller units we called "pods" or "bubbles." Work and school moved entirely online for many people, and after the school year ended, plans for summer travels and adventures faded away, as did the freedom to move about in one's town or city and places to shop, which required business owners to adapt to no-contact transactions and curbside delivery.

We faced these and many more changes—losses, really.

Of course, chief among these has been the loss of lives. In the United States alone, more than 500,000 of the over twenty-nine million people infected have died from COVID-related illness—matching what we lost in World War II and the Vietnam and Korean Wars combined—and it's not over.[1] We have lost more than many of us could have imagined.

Equally surprising has been what we have gained. I would never minimize the devastating losses of COVID-19, and especially the loss of life. Still, sitting on the front porch looking at those hills, I am keenly aware of the pandemic bringing about several things that have actually enriched my life. I have in mind unanticipated gifts such as quality time with my spouse and children; a slower life pace and the emotional space to think and be creative; occasions to reflect on my priorities, especially those relating to how I spend my time and resources; opportunities to hone a vision for living more intentionally; seeing more clearly how privileged I am; and reaffirming my duty to live in service to those who have less privilege. There's a line in a Gwendolyn Brooks poem that reads, "You are the beautiful half of a golden hurt."[2] This line captures some of the pandemic's surprises for me.

Illness

Living with Parkinson's disease can also teach you a lot about experiences that are "the beautiful half of a golden hurt," that is, simultaneously full of profound losses and surprising, invaluable gains.

For me, the gains are tied foremost to the people Parkinson's has put into my life: the doctors and therapists who treat my illness; the generous folks who lead Parkinson's organizations of

1. https://www.usnews.com/news/health-news/articles/2021-02-22/vaccine-efforts-redoubled-as-us-death-toll-draws-near-500k

2. Brooks, "To Be in Love."

which I have been fortunate to become a part; the scores of sisters and brothers who live with this wretched disease with copious amounts of grace and grit, courage and commitment, hope and joy; and the multitude of friends, colleagues, neighbors, and even strangers who, in ways large and small, encourage my kindred and me to keep up the fight, to live well, to take one day at a time, and, with our efforts, to do something good and try to tame the Parkinson's beast.

Among its many lessons, I am learning from Parkinson's that life itself is a lot like this illness. Looking out at the Frio River winding through the Texas Hill Country, it occurs to me that, for all of us, whether living with a progressive illness or not, life unfolds in ways we do not expect, its surprises both pleasant and harsh. It brings good days and difficult ones. It offers moments of joy and pain, successes and failures. It entails dreams that come true and those that get quashed. It provides occasions for deep satisfaction and weighty regret. It includes gifts that give you goosebumps and losses that break your heart.

Well-being

We assume we cannot at once lose *and* gain in the same experience, especially when our health is involved. We tend to split off and absolutize categories of experience such as illness and well-being, assuming they are incommensurable states. If one is ill, the thinking goes, then one cannot also be well.

However, as philosopher Havi Carel points out, illness and wellness can in fact go together. She notes that in our fears about becoming ill we neglect to consider the opportunities it presents for learning to live well, and perhaps better, *because of* illness, which includes things such as finding new meaning in life, reassessing personal values, resetting priorities, becoming more intentional in one's most significant relationships, accepting what one can control and what must be left alone, and perhaps most important, valuing life in the present moment.

It is as if we live on Bittersweet Lane—all of us—amid lots of beautiful halves to golden hurts.

Miraculous Things

Night

I GLANCE ONCE MORE at the digital clock on my nightstand, its lonely white numbers glowing brightly in the dark. My mind darts to my usual nocturnal questions. *How will this night unfold? Will I be fortunate enough to get six hours of sleep or will I have to settle for my more customary four to five?* I never know the answer. Either way, tomorrow morning I will pay a visit to my neurologist.

It will be a routine visit, my six-month check-up, a typical schedule for many persons with Parkinson's. Other than my ongoing struggle with sleep—a side effect of carbidopa/levodopa, a medicine that helps me move better—I feel well. As a result, I'm not anxious about this appointment.

It has not always been this way. For the first couple of years after my diagnosis, long before medication-induced insomnia moved in, I would lie in bed the night before a visit to my neurologist tossing and turning for fear of what I might hear from her mouth.

When you've never had a serious health condition, and then a single visit to the doctor slots you into a new kind of life, then you cannot help but wonder what any visit to the doctor will bring. This is life with an illness that not only lasts but gets perpetually worse—ironically, we call this *progression*.

How will my exam go? What score will I receive on the Unified Parkinson's Disease Rating Scale (UPDRS)? Will my doctor increase the dosage for any of my medications, or start me on a new one? I used to dwell on these questions and others like them. I'd watch the clock's numbers creep along toward morning with sleepy eyes kept open by a sprinting brain.

Morning

But I don't dwell on these questions anymore. A pending visit to the neurologist no longer keeps me awake at night, and here's why.

There's a line in a Paulo Coelho novel that reads, "She would consider each day a miracle—which indeed it is when you consider the number of unexpected things that could happen in each second of our fragile existences."[1] Before Parkinson's, I did not recognize as fully as I do now the fragileness of *every* day; of *every* life. Nor did I recognize each day's potential for game-changing, life-altering, and entirely unwelcome experiences. I did not live expecting unexpected things to happen unless they were good things. No, I lived as if my existence, like that of others, was more or less guaranteed; my health more or less assured if I did the right things; my life path more or less entirely mine to map out.

I lived unaware of the miracle of getting through each day, much less of having the opportunity to celebrate each day for the gift it is.

Parkinson's made me aware of this miracle, and now I wake each morning with a commitment to live differently. I can control a lot in my world, in my life, but not everything. Some things I must leave to the sphere of mystery, to the realm of unexpected things that can be as filled with joy as it is with pain. This was true before Parkinson's came so abruptly into my life, and it remains true after the fact.

I still have questions for my doctor with each appointment. My heart still grows heavier when I think about my illness

---

1. Coelho, *Veronika Decides to Die*, 209.

progressing, of what life will be like for me in twenty years. The difference now is this heaviness does not last, does not keep me up at night, and does not diminish my happiness. Nor does it hinder me from living fully. Each. Miraculous. Day.

Now, I hope I can sleep. I have an early appointment with my doctor tomorrow.

Pluck the Day

Younger Poets

ONE THING HAVING PARKINSON'S can teach you is that life is unpredictable and fleeting, two truths recently reinforced for me.

I spin on my stationary bike with the TV remote in hand, flipping mindlessly through YouTube videos as I complete my morning workout. Then, I see it—*Dead Poets Society*—and my mind dashes back to 1989, the year before I finished college, and then to an image of the late Robin Williams standing on a desk in the classroom of an all-boys boarding school in late 1950s New England.

Playing a character named John Keating, Williams is their newly hired English teacher and he brings an unconventional approach to the classroom. He gets his students to invest in the subject matter—in poetry, literature, and writing—by showing them how these literary forms can be entertaining and bring one joy, but he also shows them how literature may widen their perspectives on their lives and even prompt their courage to risk pursuing dreams with renewed vigor and steadfast resolve. In other words, a good poem, book, essay, or story has the power to change us, forever, in ways we never imagined, much less anticipated.

In another of the film's more memorable scenes, Mr. Keating asks one of his students to read from a poem they had been assigned, which opens as follows:

> *Gather ye rosebuds while ye may,*
> *Old Time is still a-flying;*
> *And this same flower that smiles today*
> *Tomorrow will be dying.*[1]

When the student finishes reading, Mr. Keating interprets its meaning by invoking the Latin phrase, carpe diem, which he says means "seize the day!" Incidentally, I learned from my friend Nick Martin, who teaches Latin, that carpe diem more accurately translates to "pluck the day." Either way, the lesson Mr. Keating wants to teach them is that because life is short, beauty is to be savored now, while we have it. We pluck the day as we might take hold of a beautiful flower, take in a sunset, or relish time spent with a cherished friend, enjoying to the fullest the gift of the present moment because life is finite and passes before we know it.

Older Poets

Earlier in the week, I had the pleasure of meeting with my close friend, Michael Adams. We are both professors at the University of Texas at Austin, and we share a love of literature, poetry, and writing. We meet regularly to talk about our interests; more accurately, we meet to talk about *my* efforts to become a better poet. Michael, you see, has served as a professor of English, as director of the prestigious Dobie Paisano Fellowship for writers, and as a leader in the University's esteemed Michener Writing Center. He's an accomplished novelist, essayist, and painter. He is also among the kindest and most interesting people I know.

As it turns out, Michael and I share something else in common. We both have Parkinson's disease. So, when we aren't talking about what I can do to become a better poet, we share our losses and wins, questions and worries, and exercise and medication

1. Herrick, "To the Virgins, to Make Much of Time."

protocols related to having this illness and keeping its progression at bay. We also cheer each other on and even laugh about some of the absolutely ludicrous things about Parkinson's.

Among the many things I appreciate about Michael, I was immediately drawn to his plainspoken ways and his resolve to speak the truth, whether in writing or in conversation. In this vein, although I doubt Michael would stand on top of a desk to underscore his point, it's not his style, I am confident that he would encourage anyone who would listen—whether they have Parkinson's or not—to pluck the day. He'd say, "Widen your perspectives on life. Indulge your passions. Muster the courage to pursue your dreams."

All of us do well to take this wisdom to heart, whatever our age or station in life. For as the poet observed,

> *Old Time is still a-flying;*
> *And this same flower that smiles today*
> *Tomorrow will be dying.*

What I Have Learned from Michael J. Fox

In the Dark

IN THE FALL OF 2016, I sat in a dark room reading Michael J. Fox's book *Lucky Man* on my Kindle as waves of anxiety rolled through me. It felt like what you expect to happen in the ocean just before a storm. A couple of months had passed since I joined the ranks of those living with Parkinson's disease before the age of fifty, the "young-onset" group, as we are called. On most days, I struggled with questions about my future and whether life could still be good for me and my family.

As many people I would come to know in this beautiful if also resilient community had done, I looked to a man I had not yet met for comfort and encouragement. He made me feel less alone in this journey I'd just begun and more hopeful about the miles ahead. Indeed, it did not take long for me to realize that the public face of Parkinson's—the Alex P. Keaton and Marty McFly and Teen Wolf of my adolescence—had a lot of wisdom to share, as well as perspective and hope in the face of adversity. To say that I relied upon Michael's infectious courage, humor, and optimistic point of view for my sanity is to overstate it only slightly. In fact, I'm not sure I would have gotten through those first weeks and months intact had it not been for *Lucky Man*, Michael's first memoir, and *Always Looking Up*, his second.[1]

Rays of Light

Here are a few things he said in those books that I read just when I needed to have nuggets of wisdom to hold onto.

- *One's dignity may be assaulted, vandalized, and cruelly mocked, but it can never be taken away unless it is surrendered.*

- *My happiness grows in direct proportion to my acceptance, and in inverse proportion to my expectations.*

- *Happiness is a decision.*

- *Acceptance doesn't mean resignation; it means understanding that something is what it is and that there's got to be a way through it.*

- *Control is illusory. No matter what university you go to, no matter what degree you hold, if your goal is to become master of your own destiny, you have more to learn.*

- And, perhaps most poignant for me to read now: *It may seem hard to believe, but it's catastrophe that offers the most promise for an even richer life. This is the gateway to the good stuff. In other words, you never truly know which way the wind is blowing until the shit hits the fan.*

We rarely associate hardships, much less catastrophe, with a gateway to something good. These experiences are, by definition, hard. They come with challenges, even struggles, monumental life shifts, and in the case of a serious medical diagnosis like PD, with lots of losses, too. But Michael is on to something here, and though I might not have believed him in those first weeks and months after my diagnosis nearly five years ago, I now know his perspective is spot on.

1. See Fox, *Lucky Man* and *Always Looking Up*. Michael's latest memoir, *No Time Like the Future*, is also full of wisdom.

Good Stuff

Just to make sure, I decided I would make a list of the "good stuff" that Parkinson's has put in my path, as a way to test Michael's way of thinking. It's not an exhaustive list, and I've compiled it without a lot of reflection, meaning I'm just writing down what comes to mind. But here I go:

- I have met extraordinary people who live with Parkinson's or who love those who do, and these folks enrich my life beyond measure.

- I appreciate life at the moment and savor each day. Today is the only day we have.

- More than ever, I care about relationships and spending meaningful time with those I love.

- Now, I notice others' pain and suffering more quickly than ever and I look for opportunities to offer support.

- I worry less about the future.

- More than ever, I value and savor deep friendships.

- Sharing my struggles, pain, questions, worries, insecurities, and simply living with more vulnerability comes much easier these days.

- No longer do I delay doing things or having experiences that interest me.

- I have learned a lot about medicine, Parkinson's research, and scientific challenges and breakthroughs.

- I have met exceptional physicians and medical staff.

- I am more compassionate and patient.

- Goodness and generosity in others stand out to me like never before.

- I take myself less seriously and laugh at myself more.

- Failure troubles me less than it used to.

- Injustice weighs on me, and I am more eager to walk in solidarity with those who are marginalized or mistreated.

- I am more content with simpler things and a less cluttered life.

- It has become clear to me that we have a health care system that provides very well for some, including me, but leaves others unattended.

- More than ever, I tell the people I'm closest to—family, friends, colleagues, and neighbors—that they are important to me, valued and loved.

So, this is my working list. I suppose I'll think of other good stuff after I post this piece, but this is what comes to mind now.

My Way Through

It's important for me to emphasize that focusing on the "good stuff" of Parkinson's does not mean having this illness is entirely good. In fact, having Parkinson's stinks. I have heard Michael say so, too. He calls it the "suckatude" of PD. But for me, trying to live each day attuned to the "good stuff" makes life better than dwelling on the "bad stuff," which robs me of the joy that comes with anything I have put on my list. As Michael says, *Happiness is a decision; and acceptance doesn't mean resignation; it means understanding that something is what it is and that there's got to be a way through it.*

My way through Parkinson's is to embrace the good it has brought me and continues to bring, especially when the shit hits the fan.

Parenting and Courage

Challenges

A CLOSE FRIEND RECENTLY told me about his feeling guilty over what he termed "a parenting fail." After his son had made a relatively small mistake, my friend spoke to him critically and without compassion and exacerbated his son's pain.

Of the many facets of life that having Parkinson's disease has prompted me to reflect on and attend to, none has garnered more of my energy than parenthood. Having Parkinson's led me, more than ever before, to discern the type of father I hope to be to my daughters, who are now ages fifteen and thirteen and who were ten and eight when I was diagnosed with PD.

When my neurologist said that he thought I had Parkinson's, literally the first words out of my mouth were, "But I have young children." Illness can feel threatening. It can also awaken you to what's at stake in your most significant relationships, bringing newfound motivation to get right the things that matter most to you or to get them as right as you can.

Insecurities

I have shared in previous chapters that in the weeks and months that followed my diagnosis, much of the fear, anxiety, and loss I experienced related to questions and concerns about how Parkinson's would affect my ability to be the father I had always imagined to Meredith and Holly. *Would I be able to do the things I'd always done with them? Would their concerns for my health get in the way of a sense of freedom and carefree life that parents want their children to have? Would Parkinson's rob us of plans we made or of new memories yet to be minted?* More haunting, *would they see me as less of a father than before?* It is hard to admit to worrying about these matters, which involved me casting my insecurities upon my children, but I have discovered that many of us diagnosed with Parkinson's earlier in life and who have younger children share similar stories of concern. Many of us ask similar questions.

Surprises

Though I could never have imagined it in those early weeks and months following my diagnosis, Parkinson's has brought a lot of beauty into my life. For example, it has fanned my desire to be a particular kind of parent. I want to be more attentive, patient, and compassionate toward my daughters, and more aware of not taking our time together for granted. Parkinson's has helped me lighten up and relax, too, and to remember what's important and what isn't.

Having Parkinson's has also helped me become more accepting of life's curveballs and more resilient as they pass, which I hope my daughters see and take note of themselves.

Give and Take

Of course, no parent gets it right every time, and I still work at being the kind of father I want to be to my daughters. I have my parenting fails. Still, I hope my daughters see regularly, especially through my failures, that life's challenges present opportunities to learn, grow, and become a better version of ourselves.

Parkinson's is a great *taker*. There's no way around that reality. It takes one's ability to walk, speak, sleep, and move, among many other things one cherishes and depends on to live well.

Period.

And yet, this *taker* bestows gifts, too, often when we least imagine it possible. I'm learning that it's okay to take this both/and approach to a life with Parkinson's: it takes and it gives; it is ugly and beautiful. For me, among its most beautiful gifts is a more informed and self-aware joy attached to being Meredith's and Holly's dad than I previously knew.

Courage

When I think of what parenting requires—its give and take, successes and failures, ugliness and beauty—a line in the John Steinbeck novel *East of Eden* comes to mind: "Perhaps it takes courage to raise children."[1]

As it does to live well with Parkinson's disease.

1. Steinbeck, *East of Eden*, 150.

A Spiritual Thing

Unfinished Spaces

"OVER THERE IS THE CATHEDRAL of St. John the Divine," I say. Peering out the large windows of our rented apartment and pointing across 110th Street, I gesture to my wife Tracey and our daughters Meredith and Holly, "Come take a look."

It's a Friday afternoon in early November and we have just arrived in New York for a long weekend. Three years have passed since my Parkinson's diagnosis, almost to the day. Sunday I will run the New York City Marathon.

Located a few blocks from Columbia University, this cathedral remains unfinished even though its construction began in the late nineteenth century. As a graduate student at Columbia in the 1990s, I occasionally went to St. John's to find solitude and to reflect on life's bigger questions: those of meaning, purpose, and hope.

Scaffolding and work crews notwithstanding, the cathedral has a long, beautiful, Gothic-style nave that still captivates me. This sanctuary—a place of refuge—draws visitors of every nation and creed. At the same time, it attracts people from a variety of religious and spiritual traditions as well as those living with more questions than answers. Seekers and skeptics, themselves unfinished and on paths of discovery, journey to this place. I suspect that, like me, many who visit long to gain more insight, perhaps to unload their burdens, and even to catch a glimpse of the divine.

Tracey and I will take our girls there on Monday, the day after the marathon.

Spiritual Things

Now, it's the evening before the marathon that grips me, when I experienced another kind of sanctuary.

Those of us running for Team Fox—120 in total and four of us with Parkinson's—gather at a Midtown restaurant for an early dinner with our families. Michael J. Fox, who has lived courageously with Parkinson's for nearly thirty years, joins us. He speaks eloquently in both humorous and poignant ways about what the Team Fox community has meant to him over the years.

Visibly moved as he looks around the room at all of us, he says, "You should see how beautiful you are," and then shares a few memories from marathons he's witnessed and speaks with joy about his foundation putting a team together each year to run.

Many of us watch with our own full hearts and moist eyes.

At one point he pauses and says, "I've been thinking about spiritual things."

He tells us that his youngest daughter's birthday sometimes falls on the day of the marathon, as it will this year, and that she was born in 2001, not long after the horrific events of 9/11. After weeks of uncertainty about there being a marathon that year, in a city carrying so much pain and with many burdens to shed, he recalls standing at his apartment window with his newborn daughter in his arms and watching crowds of marathon runners as they passed by.

He says, "I remember looking out at the people and I thought to myself . . . this is beautiful; this is what people can do and how they can overcome."

Again he pauses. Then, acknowledging that we all have our own personal pain and burdens to endure, whether because we live with Parkinson's or we love someone who does, he says, "It's the same looking out that window to look out at all of you. It means so much. I love you all. I know you are all here for your own reasons and for your own people. But we are all *our* people."

Journeys

As with any chronic illness, Parkinson's makes us journeyers. Against our will, it grabs us, disorients us, and places us on a path of discovery. There we must find our bearings and search for ways to live a full life with a disease that seeks constantly to take life away.

Like those making visits to the cathedral, we who journey with this insidious disease represent every nation, creed, and spiritual path. We also live in unfinished spaces laced with profound questions of meaning, and purpose, and hope.

What's more, we have burdens to unload. We long to find healing. Often in need of maintenance, if not repair, we require permanent scaffolding for support. For all of these reasons, and more, we need *all* our people.

I see this more vividly now.

In these unfinished spaces, with our people, I catch a glimpse of the divine.

A Letter to My Newly Diagnosed Self

It's the fall of 2016. I'm forty-eight years old, and words from a man I have only just met prompt what feels like an out-of-body experience — becoming as much an observer of what is happening to me as a participant in it. "What worries me is that I think you are in the early stages of Parkinson's," the doctor says, and everything slows as if I am watching someone else's nightmare unfold while listening to a record spinning at a sluggish speed. Things get blurry, too, and slowly the room begins to spin. I grab hold of the hard wooden chair I am sitting in, hoping to keep my breakfast down. "But I have young children . . . ," I say.

Life changed profoundly at that moment in a neurologist's office, as it does for approximately sixty thousand people each year in the United States alone who receive a Parkinson's diagnosis. A portion of them, approximately 4 percent, will be under the age of fifty. They will be said to have young-onset Parkinson's, which brings a unique set of challenges, especially because they typically will still be working and, in many cases, will still have children in the home.

Looking back on this moment nearly five years later, I feel and know so many things that I wish I could share with my newly diagnosed self. Here are a few of them.

Breathe

A Parkinson's diagnosis can feel overwhelming, and understandably so. Parkinson's disrupts life and plans for the future; and it can threaten one's sense of security, whether in terms of work and finances, relationships, or one's identity or sense of self as a healthy person. For all of these reasons, it's important to take a breath, literally and figuratively speaking. To calm down, and to begin coming to terms with Parkinson's by recalling that it's not a death sentence. (Life expectancy is nearly what it would be if you did not have Parkinson's.) Moreover, progression typically is slow, especially in younger people. You will have time to adjust to your new normal.

Consider Sharing Your Diagnosis

One of the first questions many of us have is whom we should tell we have Parkinson's. Several people I know have kept their Parkinson's diagnosis private, some for a long time. For some, there may be good reasons to keep a diagnosis private. After all, Parkinson's can come with all sorts of misperceptions, naivety, and flat-out wrong assumptions about what it will mean for a person's future. However, this silence can take a toll. You likely will have to work hard to camouflage or explain away symptoms, hiding something that has become a central part of your life.

For the first ten months after my diagnosis, I stayed silent about it. All the while, I felt disingenuous and inauthentic. It was as if I were cheating on people I care about while also being unfaithful to myself, and this became more painful than having Parkinson's. However, when I began sharing my diagnosis, I felt not only relieved but empowered to live a good life with Parkinson's. Just as importantly, being open about my condition helped me meet others living with Parkinson's. I have never regretted the decision to live openly with Parkinson's; I just wish I had begun doing so sooner.

Find Your People with Parkinson's

This brings me to the next piece of advice I would have given to my newly diagnosed self: find your people as soon as possible! One of the great gifts I have experienced because of Parkinson's is the extraordinary group of people I have met. People with Parkinson's have offered me comfort, encouragement, hope, and humor, and their support has helped me feel not only more empowered but more connected with other people, too. This connection is key. We need each other to live well with Parkinson's.

Speak to an Employment Attorney

This brings me to a practical matter: I urge you to meet with an employment attorney before going public with your diagnosis. This kind of consultation should be part of your discernment process. You will benefit from knowing your rights as well as your employer's responsibilities if you run into problematic responses. You want to make the most informed decisions you can concerning living publicly with Parkinson's, including at work. Remember that the law is on your side concerning your job and knowing as much as possible about that can provide a measure of comfort and security.

Life Can Still Be Good

Living with Parkinson's can be difficult, especially as it progresses, but life can still be good. I have found that having Parkinson's can provide opportunities for growth—personal, relational, and spiritual—and that living with Parkinson's presents opportunities for newfound meaning and deeper, more authentic relationships. Until we find a cure for Parkinson's, none of us can change our status as a person with Parkinson's. However, we can choose how we live with it, what we do with it. We decide whether it becomes a source of despair or empowerment as we live in solidarity with other people with Parkinson's, our care partners and families, and our larger networks of advocacy and support. We can boost one another and use our collective voices for making others' lives better, which makes our own lives better, too.

It's now been more than four years since my neurologist's sixteen words changed my life. At almost fifty-three years old, I now live more calmly and with a lot more knowledge about Parkinson's. I have a clearer perspective on how to experience the fullness of life, with a lot of joy and hope even amid the daily challenges that the Parkinson's beast throws down. My children are now teenagers, and we have integrated Parkinson's into our family life. It's making all of us more resilient, compassionate, and grateful for what we have, both despite Parkinson's and because of it.

Five Keys for Living Well with Illness

Keys

A RECENT VISIT TO the Lock and Key Shop on the campus of The University of Texas at Austin got me thinking about keys as they relate to a life with Parkinson's: *keys to managing our symptoms; keys to living well with this illness; keys to coping with the challenges that Parkinson's brings.* I find it helpful to remember that keys do at least a couple of things. They provide access and they offer security, letting us into spaces we desire to inhabit and keeping out what threatens us in those spaces.

When I consider the keys to living with Parkinson's, several come to mind.

- **Acceptance.** Having Parkinson's requires acknowledging the losses that come with it and accepting that life will be different going forward. A lack of acceptance or living in denial of our losses makes intrusions by things like depression, anxiety, anger, or bitterness more likely. Finding peace should be our focus, and this requires accepting our illness. But as Michael J. Fox has noted, "Acceptance doesn't mean resignation; it means understanding that something is what it is and that there's got to be a way through it."

- **A positive outlook**. Having Parkinson's stinks, no doubt. I have yet to meet a person who says they'd sign up for it. But life can still be good with Parkinson's—very good. Illness and wellness can go together. Discovering or rediscovering what brings us joy and meaning is the key. Many aspects of life can be affected by how we approach them. If we approach life with a negative, pessimistic, downer attitude or outlook, that will color our experience. But the same is true when we have a positive outlook. I try to surround myself with positive, hopeful people, too. It helps.

- **Gratitude**. I try to begin each day by asking, "What am I thankful for?" and taking note of the abundance in which I live: family, friends, work, resources, health (yes, despite Parkinson's), interests, talents, the Parkinson's community, and more. Cicero said, "Gratitude is not only the greatest of virtues, but the parent of all others." It's stunning how helpful it can be to start the day in a posture of thanksgiving and gratitude.

- **Community**. Another key may be found in identifying the family members, friends, colleagues, and neighbors you can rely on and who offer support and encouragement. I am convinced that how we fare in a life with Parkinson's, really, in any life, is directly related to the community we have around us. We cannot do this illness alone or in isolation. Many of us have discovered this the hard way. Find your people as quickly as you can, lean on them, invite them to lean on you, and you'll likely find it helps you feel better and live with greater satisfaction and calm.

- **Education**. "Knowledge is power," observed Francis Bacon, the sixteenth-century English philosopher, recognizing that with greater awareness and understanding comes greater control. Learning as much as we can about the illness with which we live is a key to living well. Greater understanding helps us not only gain more resources for managing Parkinson's, but it makes us feel better and helps us live as if we have more power over Parkinson's, which we do.

Five More Keys for Living Well with Illness

IN THE LAST CHAPTER, I wrote about some of the keys for me to live well with Parkinson's: *acceptance, a positive outlook, gratitude, community, and education.* Here, I want to share a few more keys that give me access to spaces I want to inhabit in a life with Parkinson's and keep out what threatens me in those spaces.

More Keys

When I consider the keys to living with Parkinson's, several come to mind.

- **Discipline**. I find that being disciplined in a life with Parkinson's is a key to managing it. I'm talking about discipline concerning things like exercise, medication protocols, seeing doctors and other care team members (physical therapists, speech therapists, and counselors), spending time with running partners, writing partners, our sisters and brothers in the Parkinson's community, and others who enrich our lives. For me, attention to these matters makes a big difference in how I feel, physically, emotionally, and spiritually. But the key is that I have to be disciplined in my efforts. I have to commit to these practices and stay with them. Otherwise, I lose the benefits they offer.

- **Goals**. Parkinson's is the great thief. It steals many things from us that we want and need for a good life. Among the most valuable things it can steal from us, but which we can also protect from its grasp, are our goals for the future. I find that many people who live with Parkinson's assume their previous goals (and the dreams linked to them) are unreachable and that formulating and pursuing new goals is a waste of time. Nothing could be further from the truth. We can still pursue our goals and plan to work toward new ones. So get going on that if you're not already working on it. Keep aiming for what brings you joy, meaning, purpose, and a sense of accomplishment. Adjusting goals is fine—we all have to do this sometimes, whether we have Parkinson's or not. The point is that having goals is part and parcel of being human, so don't give up on pursuing your goals.

- **Purpose**. Another key I will mention is that all of us need purpose in life—all of us. And while it's true that life becomes more challenging with Parkinson's, there are still many things that we can do that give us a sense of purpose and, as important, that may contribute to others' well-being and positive outlook along with ours. I'm thinking of things like reaching out to others in the Parkinson's community and offering to help them with what they may need: a ride to an exercise class or support group, or a doctor's visit. A phone call to someone who is struggling with anxiety or depression. Allowing a care partner for a person with Parkinson's (PwP) to have a couple of hours of respite. We can also send emails, texts, or cards to those who might benefit from knowing they are thought of and that we are sending well wishes (and who doesn't benefit from receiving these kind gestures?). We can raise money for Parkinson's support services or research. We can also help educate others and raise awareness of Parkinson's and needed resources for support. If we have a purpose we are happier, more settled, and more satisfied with our lives.

- **Humor**. The comedian Steve Martin once noted that "A day without sunshine is like, you know, night." This brings me to humor. For me, a key to managing Parkinson's is finding ways to laugh every day, including, at times, laughing at or with Parkinson's. Having Parkinson's is not funny per se (no one wants to have it) but it does come with moments of humor. For example, when my daughters were young, I was grumpy with one of our dogs because he was barking out the window at another dog, and one of my girls looked at me and said, "Daddy, be nice to him; he has Barkinson's disease." This moment and countless others like it have been a balm for me, and for my family, that provides relief from the pain that adjoins a life with Parkinson's. Also, while I am not all that funny, my wife and children are extremely funny! So my advice is to find the funny people in your life and spend as much time with them as you can.

And remember Steve Martin's wisdom.

Sandcastles

Building

ON A RECENT FAMILY trip to the coast, I started to think about sandcastles. Our family excursions to the beach always include building sandcastles, a practice that began when my children were very young and which involves three generations of family members.

Sometimes, the sandcastles we build are small and modest. Other times, they get more elaborate. Our creations also include more than sandcastles: animals, faces of famous people, and a Texas Longhorns logo, for example. Part of the fun is seeing who can come up with the most creative or outlandish idea, and then bring it to life in the sand.

Tides

Whatever we build is gone within a few hours. The tides roll in and wash it away, mixing it back into the ocean's floor where it awaits another day's creative efforts. But our knowledge that everything will be washed away never gives us pause, much less prevents us from hauling our shovels and tools and buckets to the beach, spending significant time on our hands and knees crawling around each other, and building what we want.

The act of making something meaningful to us, and doing so with the people we love most, has inherent value. Sharing fun and joyful experiences, despite their fleeting nature, is something we willingly engage in, year after year. Walt Whitman wrote, "I tramp a perpetual journey." Building sandcastles reminds me of why and how the perpetual journey matters so much.

Rebuilding

Our lives are like sandcastles. We build them and then parts of us get washed away by the tides of life. Some tides are gentle and warm, others are jarring and cold. Either way, after they wash in and out we rebuild and continue tramping a perpetual journey. Then, eventually, the tides wash in and out again, and we repeat the process once more.

After my daughters constructed a monument to our home state in the sand, they took a walk on the beach together and I wrote this poem:

Sandcastles

The blue beach house sits in a row
With six others, all of a different color,
Forming a rainbow on the shore,
Rain or shine.

A thin salty film clings to ocean-facing windows,
Humid breezes move across a wooden porch
Bringing familiar beachy smells,
A couple of seagulls glide overhead and squawk.

We first came here when
Our daughters were four and two,
When we sat at the water's edge
Making sandcastles,

Sandcastles

Walking the beach in search of seashells,
Flying kites, sharing picnic lunches,
Running toward the steel
Pushcart carrying lemon ices.

Now teenagers,
They make plans with one another—
To drive golf carts, go for walks, and
Search for boys acceptable to me.

Sitting at the water's edge,
I linger in my memories and smile,
Making sandcastles
On my own.

Riding the Wave

Shaking

I FLOAT ON MY BACK in the green glassy lake, feet sticking out of the water and toes gripping the rubber tread on the slick fiberglass board. My teenage daughter sits on the boat near four of her friends and their dads. One dad is perched tall in the driver's seat. The other dad sits on the stern, arm cocked, ready to toss the rope.

It's my first time trying to wake surf behind a ski boat. I am usually the one driving, pulling my daughter and watching her pop a giant smile when effortlessly catching the perfect wave. Today, I float in the water, courtesy of a black life jacket, hoping to stand on the board.

My daughter tosses me the rope. My heart beats faster. My body begins shaking slightly, as if it's a cold winter's day, but it's only a Parkinson's adrenaline response, which I know well.

Reflecting

My mind drifts for a moment, harking back five years to when I heard those life-altering words from a doctor, "You have Parkinson's disease," and assumed my life was all but over. I thought, too, of my nearly one year of hiding and suffering in silence.

I never imagined I'd be learning to wake surf five years later, and much less that life would be richer than ever before in certain ways: the generous people I have met because of Parkinson's; the deep reflections on values, priorities, and perspectives now shaped by a chronic, progressive illness that does not relent; that an awful disease could make me a better father, partner, colleague, and friend.

"Are you okay, Daddy?" my daughter asks.

I give her a thumbs up and blow her a kiss before going through a checklist of things to do.

Let the boat pull me up. Keep my knees bent. Transfer my weight once I'm up and out of the water. Square my shoulders with the wake. Let the wave do the work.

Failing

Four times, I try and fail. What feels like a gallon of lake water shoots up my nose as I struggle to stand and then to balance myself on the small, unforgiving board. My heart beats faster and my body quivers as my daughter looks on.

"Give me one more shot," I say to the driver. "I think I know what I'm doing wrong."

The driver pulls the boat close to me and the other dad throws out the rope.

"The fifth time's the charm," I say, before rehearsing my checklist a final time.

Surfing

I give a thumbs up. The driver hits the throttle and the boat's engine revs, pulling me forward. The wake quickly grows tall as I plow for a few feet and then pop out of the water and stand on the board, knees slightly bent, shoulders mostly square to the boat's tall wake, a little wobbly but surfing, as I did as a boy in the green Atlantic.

My daughter yells, "There you go, Dad!"

I pop a giant smile as I ride the wave and look to the sky.

Darkness and Light

Midnight

I SIT IN MY CAR outside Dell Children's Hospital, just a stone's throw away from my home in Austin, Texas. Rain falls in heavy sheets and the dark sky lights up every few seconds as deep-toned thunder rolls in. It's almost midnight. Only a few hospital rooms stacked on multiple floors still have lights glowing.

I hope the children are not frightened by the storm.

My wife and I brought our daughter to the emergency room after she experienced severe abdominal pain that did not relent. Due to COVID-19 protocols, only one parent can accompany a child inside the ER, so after providing insurance information and checking my daughter in, I go sit in the car, periodically texting with my wife and daughter as we all await the doctor's arrival.

Eight excruciating hours later, which included multiple exams and imaging, we learn that my daughter's condition is nothing serious and should abate quickly.

Daybreak

Letting out a deep sigh and rubbing my heavy, red, slightly burning eyes, a poem I wrote recently comes to mind:

The River

Fresh sunlight
Touches the shallow river,
Its waters flowing toward
Places not yet known.
A warm June breeze blows,
Waking brushy hilltops
Dry from hot
Spring days and nights.

A mourning dove
Sits on a rock and coos,
Calling out to the waters
Snaking through tall banks.

Life unfolds as the river flows,
With waters tranquil and troubled.
What lies around the bend
We do not know.

New Day

We get in the car and start the one-mile trip home as the new day's sun reveals a now clear sky. Pulling out of the hospital parking lot, fighting off sleep, I notice one hospital room, its light still burning from the night before. My mind drifts to the child and the loved ones surely gathered in the room. A pediatric hospital is a place of long days and sometimes longer nights. It is a place of worry, anger, disbelief, and heartache, a place where both good news and bad news are delivered, where everyone waits and hopes.

I swallow hard as we pull away from the hospital.

Approaching our home, I see the dim glow of a single light, which we left on in case our other teenaged daughter awakened before we returned home. I look momentarily at her bedroom window, where she still sleeps, and then peer into the rearview mirror, where my wife has our younger daughter tucked under her chin. I pull into our driveway, park, and take from my pocket a tablet of carbidopa/levodopa, my Parkinson's wonder drug, which my sleepless and stiff body knows I am late taking.

Life feels more precious *and* delicate than it did just a few hours before.

Five Years

An Anniversary

I AWAKEN EARLY, AROUND 5 AM, as I do most mornings. It's quiet and the city lies still as I turn on the coffee pot, let our three dogs outside, and place food in their bowls. It will be another hour before my wife Tracey gets up for her marathon training run, and a bit longer until our girls wake up and get ready for school.

The day before, Tracey reminded me in a brief text that "Tomorrow is your anniversary." Yes, today marks five years since a doctor I had just met uttered sixteen life-changing words: *What worries me is that I think you are in the early stages of Parkinson's disease.*

I have written a lot about the five years since that day. One may read through the various stories on in this book to glimpse facets of my journey from diagnosis, to secrecy, to acceptance, and eventually, to finding meaning, purpose, and hope in a new kind of life.

Today

This morning, after taking my daughter to school, I will meet for coffee with my friend Gary, who also lives with Parkinson's, and we will talk about things we care about, share how we are faring, and surely have a few laughs. Gary is one of the many gifts Parkinson's has brought into my life.

From there, I will go to campus and meet with colleagues and students and generous donors about work we all love and to which we happily devote our lives and resources. After work, I will meet my pal Jordan for a beer, and we will do what friends do: talk about mutual interests, our families, our work, the stuff of life.

Then, I'll spend the evening with my wife and two daughters, sharing a meal, talking about our day, checking in regarding school, homework, and friendships. Finally, we will rest knowing we've done our best by this day. After five years, we now know and accept that tomorrow Parkinson's will bring both challenges and gifts. And we'll wake up ready to start again.

Five Years

Five years of living with what my diagnosing neurologist, Dr. T, called "a new family member" has brought about some of the darkest moments of my life but also many more of the brightest. Those years were ones of friendships and community, marathons, efforts to raise awareness and funding for Parkinson's research, and to offer education. In those five years, a renewed commitment to and passion for living each day to the fullest took hold. I have learned to live daily with an illness that will never define me but which guides me and provides meaning, purpose, perspective, and even joy that I never could have imagined possible as those sixteen words left Dr. T's mouth.

Journeys

A lot fills my heart's space this morning. The following poem, written a few months ago, captures some of what I think and feel, and importantly, some of what I want others to know, wherever they may be on their journeys, whether with Parkinson's or other challenges thrown their way.

Healing

Happiness does not require a cure.
Neither does feeling at peace with illness.
Otherwise, I am sentenced to discontentment,
Gripped by anxiety or resentment.

If happiness presumes wellness
I forego each day's openings—for
Passion and learning, significance and purpose,
For indescribable joy with those I love.

Looking at the horizon for a cure
Must not take my eyes away
From beautiful vistas and
Sacredness before me.

Illness teaches this.
I am also learning that,
While it may surprise us,
Healing can precede cures.

Remembering Our Strengths

Naivety

I RECEIVED A DIAGNOSIS of young-onset Parkinson's disease five years ago, at the age of forty-eight, and I immediately became pre-occupied with becoming disabled. Among my greatest concerns was that I would quickly lose the ability to do things I enjoyed, such as swimming and biking with my kids, working out at the gym, traveling with my family, and teaching at my university. Anxious that I would have to stop doing any of these things, or other things that bring me joy and meaning, I remember asking my doctor to assure me that I would dance at my daughters' weddings (they were aged ten and eight at the time), to which she responded, "I am confident you will."

I now realize that this expectation was naïve on more than one front. My daughters might not want to get married or have a wedding. Nevertheless, as often happens with a Parkinson's diagnosis, anxiety took over my worldview and had its say for nearly a year; but at the end of that long year, I'm glad to tell you my stress started to wane, for three reasons.

First, I got to know numerous people living with Parkinson's who remained active and doing what they loved for many years

—even decades—after their diagnosis. Second, I shifted my focus away from an unknown future and toward celebrating the gift of today, and I started to consider what I *have* more than what I might someday *lose*. Third, I began to learn from those who live with disabilities, who may face obstacles to doing certain things but who also learn to mitigate those challenges and, often, discover new talents and opportunities. I started seeing disability through a lens of strengths, not merely of deficits.

Ability

What I was naïve about is just how much *ability* those who have disabilities possess. Those living with disabilities offer distinct insights and perspectives; they exhibit resilience-born wisdom, as well as discipline and a strong work ethic. Because persons with disabilities must constantly adapt to their surroundings, they also bring creativity, agility, persistence, openness, forethought, and capacity for solving problems. These strengths are admirable, attractive, and they serve anyone and any community well.

Similar to my naivety regarding my daughters getting married, I was naïve about those who live with disabilities, or who, like me, might become disabled someday. I now recognize that we are strong, unique, and we enhance the common good. We may have disabilities but these need not define us, nor do they limit our potential in every way. Remembering our strengths and opportunities helps me feel less anxious about the future and more empowered for living with Parkinson's today.

··· 24 ···

More Mayo, Please

Travelers

THE ATRIUM, WITH ITS tall ceiling and a vast amount of glass, allows light to come in from several directions as a middle-aged woman sits at a shiny black grand piano and plays an airy tune. Dressed in hospital scrubs, she has just finished her twelve-hour shift as a nurse. I'm told that she and a few other staff members are known to conclude many of their shifts in this way.

She plays a Mozart piece, one that my daughter sometimes plays at home, while scores of people pass by. Some use canes or walkers. Others roll by in wheelchairs. Others wear prosthetic devices on their legs, feet, arms, or hands. Just down the hallway from the piano, one sees the store where wigs, breast prostheses, and compression clothing are available for purchase.

I look over at Vanessa, my talented filmmaker friend, who scans the room with pursed lips. We stand on hallowed ground and watch sacred acts unfold.

We are in Rochester, Minnesota, at the renowned Mayo Clinic. People come here from all over the country and the world because they are sick and have a need for healing, and often they arrive after unsuccessful stopovers in other hospitals and treatment centers. It's a destination, a site for medical pilgrims, including patients and providers, and a place where people's deepest hopes are realized and can also remain unfulfilled.

Healers

We have come here to interview Dr. Rodolfo Savica, a neurologist and movement disorder specialist whose focus is on young-onset Parkinson's disease. He has unconventional takes on this illness with which I and many others live, even viewing it as a different disease than typical, later-onset Parkinson's. He'll be featured in a documentary film that Vanessa and I are making.

One needs only a few moments in the doctor's presence to discover that his knowledge and wisdom as a researcher are matched by his passion for clinical work and by a tireless effort to help his patients feel better and live better with this illness.

He came to Mayo more than a decade ago from Italy, his sole purpose being to hone his calling as a healer, to do his life's work. "I fell in love with the basal ganglia," he says, "and I deeply value the teamwork approach at Mayo. All of us work together to support patients . . . to support one another." As Tolstoy noted of those in the healing arts, "They satisf[y] that eternal human need for hope of relief, for sympathy, and that something should be done, which is felt by those who are suffering."[1]

Vanessa and I spend the day with Dr. Savica and a kind woman named Susan, who serves as one of Mayo's public relations and media consultants and who also speaks a lot about their core values and commitment to teamwork. Her kindness, dry sense of humor, and Midwestern hospitality must enrich many lives. Early the next morning we leave Rochester for Minneapolis, where we will change planes, fly to Portland, Oregon, and continue work on the documentary.

---

1. Tolstoy, *War and Peace*, Part 9, Ch. 16.

Dreamers

While on this flight I begin thinking about how, as a society, we tend to tuck illness away, keeping it out of sight and thus out of mind, as we focus on fitness and shun aging. We do this tucking for a variety of reasons, including out of deep-seated fear and even feelings of shame over bodies that deteriorate over time. For nearly a year, I tucked away my own diagnosis with Parkinson's.

What I realize is how much I wish there were more Mayo Clinics in the world, places where cutting-edge science and medicine shape offers of care, yes, but equally, where airy atriums warm what can be experienced as cold, impersonal, clinical spaces; where having a wig store is highly valued and oddly provides a feeling of comfort; and where people dare to extend kindness toward strangers simply because all of us are human and all of us struggle.

I also wish that more people who face a serious illness or who companion a loved one facing it could have a Mayo-like experience, with its sacred beauty, a nurse playing Mozart, an ebullient doctor who speaks of his love of the basal ganglia. I wish more of us could experience light coming into our lives, despite our illness, along with other unanticipated gifts of life, love, and hope. I wish we all had that Mayo teamwork vibe where we receive treatment.

After landing in Minneapolis, the Delta flight attendant greets us over the PA system, "We thank you for flying with us, and for all of you receiving treatment at Mayo, take care of yourselves and know that we wish you well."

When she finishes, I turn up the volume as Mozart plays through my earbuds.

The Button

Hands

BEFORE PARKINSON'S, MY FINGERS and hands worked better than they do now. I don't mean to boast, but, for example, I used to be able to change my girls' diapers with one hand. My ability developed over the course of weeks and, out of necessity, was honed over a longer period of time.

My wife Tracey and I produced two daughters—two *active* daughters, Meredith and Holly, now ages sixteen and fourteen—who treated a diaper change like a pit stop in the Indianapolis 500. Parked on the changing table, they kept their engines revved up, and the pit crew had mere seconds to get the job done.

When I was the sole member of the diaper change pit crew, one of my hands served as brakes, keeping those revved up little bodies from speeding away, while the other hand accomplished the diaper change. Being a bit competitive, I started timing myself; and by the time Holly was toilet trained, I could do a full pit stop, one-handed, consistently in less than thirty seconds. My best time was twenty-five seconds. Wipes included!

The Button

Now, fourteen years later, I struggle some days with buttoning my shirt sleeves, especially my right one, as my dexterity in my left hand comes and goes. My fingers don't move like they used to. PD has affected me most on my left side, and I'm left-handed.

The Button represents several things for me. First, it reminds me that Parkinson's doesn't get better. It's a progressive illness and the difficulty I have with buttoning my right shirt sleeve will only increase. As I dress for work each morning, I face that hard reality.

On the other hand, the Button also reminds me that, in many cases, those of us who struggle with physical challenges can find work-arounds. We are a resourceful bunch! I know numerous people living with Parkinson's who avoid buttons altogether, opting for different types of shirts, and who wear slip-on shoes so they don't have to tie shoelaces, and who shave only with an electric razor.

More importantly, the Button reminds me to practice self-compassion and acceptance. By self-compassion I mean the need to give ourselves a break from the pressure to always have ourselves put together, fronting out with our most impeccable appearance, the tidiest and most pristine versions of ourselves. Perhaps the most telling thing about my daughters and their pit stops is that they could not have cared less if their naked butts were visible to the world. There are lessons to be learned from that, just as there are from buttons on clothing.

Helpers

My buddy Dan Stultz also lives with Parkinson's and has for fourteen years. He gave up practicing medicine a few years ago but he still shows proficiency with a chainsaw and bulldozer. Dan often says that when it comes to living with Parkinson's, "It is what it is." Accepting it and doing the best we can, its challenges notwithstanding, is our choice to make. We are a lot happier when we do this. We live more at peace. We are also more productive.

Dan also reminded me recently that, eventually, everyone deals with physical or other kinds of challenges. Everyone. Life is what it is. Parkinson's just happens to be Dan's and my challenge, and maybe yours.

Sometimes, when I peer into an imagined future, I think about the time when I will have to ask for help buttoning my shirt, or with other basic tasks of daily life, whether from Tracey or from Meredith or Holly. "Will this be the year?" I ask myself.

Honestly, though I keep trying to delay it, whenever that year comes, I'll be okay with it. I'll be ready to ask for the help I need from Tracey, Meredith, Holly, and others in my life; and I will be eager to help them too if they have the need. This is just what we do.

It's also possible that as Meredith and Holly button my shirt sleeves, I'll time them.

I might even try to speed away.

26

A Bucket and a Pot of Gold

Bucket

My friend Dale calls Parkinson's his "Bucket of Shit," or "Bucket" for short. He and I are close to the same age, and he's had Bucket since 2015, a year or so longer than I have.

It's St. Patrick's Day, and I'm with Dale in his hometown of Chicago. My family and I are here for me to work, but also to visit Dale and his family, other friends, and to tour colleges for my daughter Meredith, while she and her younger sister Holly are on Spring Break.

We're also going to see the Eagles on Saturday night, compliments of Dale, just as I turn fifty-four!

Friendship

Over breakfast, Dale and I talk about his work running a large company, including some of the business challenges they faced last year and his hopes for the coming fiscal quarter. He talks about his awesome wife Hope and their eight-year-old twins, and I talk about my awesome wife Tracey and our girls—the things proud and grateful middle-aged husbands and fathers talk about when they get together.

We also share what symptoms currently trouble us the most: for Dale, it's fatigue and slowness; for me, trouble sleeping and stiffness. And we discuss the latest research and treatment for Parkinson's, the new documentary film that I'm making with my film-maker friend, Vanessa, and some of the hopes I have for PD Wise.

My friendship with Dale is a source of great happiness and meaning for me, not to mention laughter and fun. Our time together enriches my life.

Later this week, Tracey, Meredith, Holly, and I will visit other friends in the Chicagoland area, people who also grace our lives with generosity and love, and whom we know only because we share the Bucket: Bill and Heidi, Abbe, and, I hope, Jimmy and Cherryl. We will surely talk about some of the things Dale and I talked about. This is what happens when those with PD get together. But we will mostly talk about other things we care about, find meaning in, aspire to, celebrate, puzzle over, struggle with, and search for—the stuff friends share.

Pot of Gold

Looking out of Dale's office and seeing the freshly dyed-green Chicago River, my mind flashes to one of the folktales associated with the worldwide celebration of Patrick, Ireland's patron saint.

The story involves rainbows, leprechauns, and pots of gold. Leprechauns, you'll recall, are small, grumpy people who enjoy playing tricks on you and are thus to be avoided. Solitary by nature, they live alone and work repairing the shoes of Irish fairies, who pay the leprechauns with golden coins that they collect in large pots. Supposedly, their pots of gold are found at the end of a rainbow, but because you can never locate the end of a rainbow, the only way to get the gold is to catch the leprechaun.

Before Parkinson's, I never believed in leprechauns or fairies.

Nor did I imagine that a bucket of shit could pair with a pot of gold.

27

Jumping to the Skies

Physics

HARRY SITS ACROSS THE round table in my campus office just after lunchtime. A quiet man with a large brain and a similar-sized heart, his career as a physicist has put him in the company of Nobel laureates and garnered him invitations to speak around the globe about his own work. You'd never know it, though, because he's as unassuming as he is smart.

Harry is my neighbor and friend. He has dropped by my office to tell me about Al, a colleague of his just diagnosed with Parkinson's.

We speak about Al, touch on life in our university, and update one another on our families. Then, I mention how excited my daughter Meredith is to take physics next year in school. "She's long been bookish but, until last year, found math more difficult than her other subjects," I say. That's when her teacher, Sean, broadened her mathematical mind. He also helped ease her anxiety and build her confidence in ways no previous math teacher had. "Sean met her where she was and helped her find and flip the switch. Then, the light came on," I say. "She began to think of math differently, to approach it in a new way, and to see herself as a mathematician. It was then that she got the physics bug."

Harry's smile raises his kind eyes as he begins telling me of his own story with math. "Growing up in Louisiana, I was a middling student in high school. Then, a teacher named Dessie McKenzie Tucker introduced me to geometry and to different ways of approaching math," he says. "I learned to do a few proofs and I thought, 'I'm pretty good at this, and it's fun,' and I kept working at it and learning."

Harry hasn't stopped. Now in his eighties, he continues to write academic papers and advise students, and shows no signs of letting up.

Parkinson's

Our conversation reminds me of something Robert Frost anecdotally observed, namely, that "There are two kinds of teachers: the kind that fills you with so much quail shot that you can't move, and the kind that just gives you a little prod behind and you jump to the skies." Then, I begin thinking about my Parkinson's teachers; those who've prodded me, often without knowing, to live my best life with this illness.

There are physicians and scientists like Drs. McCarty, Peckham, Ondo, Okun, Dorsey, Savica, and others; and celebrities who have written books or given interviews about life with Parkinson's: Michael J. Fox being at the top of the list. I continue to learn from their insights and wisdom, which helps me live better with this illness and, I hope, to support others as well.

The understanding gleaned from additional teachers is where I linger, those also who walk their own Parkinson's path. There's Dan, who looks "the Animal" in the eye daily and tells it it's not going to win that day. There's Ethan, who so naturally shares his quick wit and good humor, reminding me that joy and laughter can live beside loss and tears. There's also Keri, whose determination to learn as much about the latest research and treatment options and to share these findings empowers me and others, building resilience and resolve. And there's Michael, whose artistic eye sees with degrees of clarity and precision that I can only dream of, and who lives amid daily challenges with admirable kindness and grace.

Jumping to the Skies

Each of these teachers, along with others, has met me where I am and helped broaden my mind. They've all prodded me with their personal examples, with their ways of being and relating, and in the more challenging moments with this devious disease, I remember what they have helped me discover about humor, wisdom, benevolence, decency, and resolve. I remember what they have helped me discover about myself, which helps ease anxiety and spurs confidence for taking Parkinson's on.

"There are two kinds of teachers: the kind that fills you with so much quail shot that you can't move, and the kind that just gives you a little prod behind and you jump to the skies."

Like Meredith and Harry, I'm grateful for my teachers.

Perhaps I can introduce them to Harry's colleague Al.

Commencement

Gathering

IT'S A SATURDAY MORNING, the day of commencement, and I stand before the crowd gathered to honor E4Texas graduates. Offered by the Texas Center for Disability Studies, whose home is in the Steve Hicks School of Social Work, where I am a professor, E4Texas provides coaching in life skills and job training and placement assistance for high school graduates with intellectual or developmental disabilities. I have the honor of giving the keynote address for this auspicious occasion.

Speaking

Well, here you are, graduates of E4Texas. You've done the hard work. You're ready for jobs in childcare, personal care, and as paraprofessionals in education. You are going to be supporting others and making their lives better. I know of no higher calling nor of more meaningful work. So I want to start by saying congratulations. Congratulations to you, your families, and other supporters who are here. This is a big day. So, graduates, please stand if you are able, turn around, and let your people see you and celebrate you.

Commencement marks a beginning. All of you are beginning a new phase of your lives as you enter the workforce and make your contributions to others' lives. While that's a great privilege, it also comes with great responsibility.

As graduates of the E4Texas program, you have embraced this responsibility. You have worked hard to develop your understanding of yourselves and of meaningful work. I suspect there have been some challenging moments along the way—there are always these moments in school and life—and you have shown resilience, perseverance, and strength. You made it, and you are ready to meet the challenges that come with more independence and adulthood.

I want to offer a little advice for you to think about as you celebrate your accomplishments, as you prepare for your working future, and especially as you face challenges ahead.

But before I offer that advice, you should know where it comes from.

It comes from my own experiences with facing challenges, and specifically, the challenge of being diagnosed with young-onset Parkinson's disease five years ago. As someone who now faces a future with a disability—as a person you might be helping someday—I think a lot about facing challenges and what it takes to meet them and live well.

Here's my first piece of advice. Remember to stop and smell the roses. By that I mean take time to enjoy your life and your accomplishments. Don't dwell on the past. Don't live too much in the future. Focus on today. The future does not exist. Today is what we have. Live each day to the fullest. Work on being happy. Don't sweat the small stuff. Stop and smell the roses.

My second piece of advice is to remember that while challenges will come, you can meet those challenges and grow from them. Life's hardships are the road map to wisdom. We grow, mature, and improve most when we struggle and strain. It might not always feel that way, but it's true. Remind yourselves of this as often as you can. Remind yourselves that you are smart, courageous, resilient, and strong. You are ready to meet the challenges that come your way. You are ready to thrive.

Here's my last piece of advice. Remember your people. You have people in your life who love you, cheer for you, and who will be there for you when you need them most. Some of those people are here today, others are here in spirit, but you are never alone and you need not face your challenges by yourselves. Lean on your people, just as you want them to lean on you. We all need our people. Remember this.

I then tell the story of Cooper, a young boy who stuttered, and his father. I've written about them in chapter 3.

Sharing

The room is filled with smiling, satisfied faces and with postures that seem to reflect more confidence than they did when this class began its work eighteen months ago. My colleagues and their teams have, once again, helped young people with disabilities mature, grow, and learn skills and dispositions that will set them up for success in life. I know the students have helped their teachers grow, too.

There is also a palpable sense of solidarity derived from mutual experiences of joy and pain, familial love, shared aspirations, and hard-fought dreams. These graduates exemplify courage and resolve, perseverance and persistence. Most importantly, they bear witness to the immutable power of a community whose members believe in each other and root for each other.

As I end my speech, with my left thumb twitching, my elbow stiff and bent, and my hand slightly drawn, Dorothy Day's words come to mind. "We have all known the long loneliness and we have learned that the only solution is love and that love comes with community."[1]

1. Day, *Long Loneliness*, 286.

.... 29 ....

The Long Hallways of Illness

Treatment

ELLA, MY FATHER'S KIND and seasoned nurse, pats him on the shoulder and says, "Last one," as his weekly chemotherapy session begins. Ella's tone is both resolute and celebratory. Her words mark a moment of hope.

We won't know for several weeks whether this is indeed my dad's last round of chemo. His doctors, though positive and cautiously optimistic, cannot say definitively what the next steps will be until my dad finishes radiation in a couple of weeks and then waits four to six more weeks before having another round of scans. That's when we will know whether the growth on his lower esophagus, located near his stomach, has been eradicated or at least shrunk sufficiently for him to have surgery to remove it.

"Surgery is the goal," his oncologist says, having stopped by to check on my dad. "And the plan will be to refer him to a terrific team at Emory; they do this surgery all the time." He pauses, looks at me, and says, "If he were my dad, that's where I'd want him to go."

Ironically, in two days my older daughter will visit Emory University as we take our first steps into the world of college tours.

Memories

My father's drip continues, dropping powerful medicines into his body. While killing cancer they also make him nauseous, zap his energy, and lead to nights of fractured sleep, among other disruptions.

He drifts off into sleep, a blanket over his legs and a recliner wrapping his now slender body.

I sit at his side and watch him sleep for a brief time, and then my mind drifts to a number of memories we've shared—his coaching me in sports throughout childhood, riding dirt bikes with him urging me on, us going to the Indianapolis 500 when I was in my twenties, him smiling and giving me two thumbs up as I walked up the aisle of the chapel at Princeton University, having received my PhD and eager to embark on an academic career.

In these moments, all of them embossed in my memory, he gifted me support and encouragement, urged me to dream big, work hard, and believe good things would follow. He guided me while also releasing me to live my own life, travel my own path, and, as we used to say, "Be my own man."

He was and is my hero, and for a long time, a part of me believed he was almost invincible.

Moments

His nurse returns one last time just as the last plastic bag of medicine drips dry. My dad says, "Even though this is my last scheduled treatment I'm coming back next week to see all of you. Thank you for all you've done for me." Ella says, "Mr. Cole, you're always welcome. We won't give you any medicine next week but you can visit anytime."

My dad stands up from the recliner, smooths out the tape covering the gauze Ella applied to his forearm where the IV was placed, and walks through double doors and down a long hallway toward the lobby, where he will check in for his radiation treatment.

I walk beside him, offering support and encouragement, seeking for words to help keep him strong and dreaming big, urging him to believe good things will happen as his cancer story unfolds, just as his doctors have indicated is their belief.

Heroes

As we sit together in the lobby, watching other cancer patients and their people come and go, I have an even deeper sense of the weight of illness. I especially feel the weight of watching someone you love living with the disruptions, discomfort, and disorienting effects of illness, which makes me think of my mother, my wife and children, and myself.

I think, too, of all of us who are on journeys with illness ourselves—Parkinson's, MS, cancer, diabetes, and so many more—and those of us who will be. I think of our heroes, our dreams, and our tendency to live as if those we love—and maybe we ourselves—are almost invincible.

The radiology technician walks over and says, "Mr. Cole, we are ready for you." My dad and I stand up and I walk with him and the technician to the double doors that open to another long hallway and end at the radiation room.

My dad looks over at me and says, "Let's do this."

I give him two thumbs up and watch him walk away.

Stepping Outside the Cave

Between Friends

IT'S EARLY MORNING, AND my friend Michael and I sit at a corner table inside Jo's Coffee, where we meet weekly. Our respective journeys with Parkinson's disease intersected a couple of years ago. A mutual love of books, writing, teaching, and paradox has kept us on an already well-worn path of friendship that may best be characterized by a line in a Steinbeck novel, "I got you to look after me, and you got me to look after you, and that's why."[1]

After nearly an hour of conversation, including our challenges, frustrations, celebrations, and joys, I tell Michael about a song my daughter Meredith wrote a couple of weeks earlier. A lover of music and singing, Meredith and four friends who met in a summer music program formed a band—Sigmund Floyd. The band's first song is titled "Plato's Cave," and Meredith penned the song's lyrics.

I play a recording for Michael.

1. Steinbeck, *Of Mice and Men*, 15.

Plato's Cave

How can you describe the sun
If you've only seen the cave
Shadows bouncing on the walls
Never seen the light of day
Break your chains and step outside
See the world with your own eyes
They won't believe the things you say
If they only know the cave
Color means nothing if you've never seen
Pain means nothing if you never bleed
What you do and where you go
Dictates everything you know
Sound means nothing if you've never heard
Language means nothing if you can't read words
To see the world you need to be brave
Maybe we're all prisoners in Plato's cave
If you've only seen the darkness
How do you know that you aren't blind
Living life with your back to the fire
What's there to lose when it's time to die
I have loved and I have lost
I've had to learn and I've had to grow
There's so little that I've seen
There's so little that I know
Color means nothing if you've never seen
Pain means nothing if you never bleed
What you do and where you go
Dictates everything you know
Sound means nothing if you've never heard
Language means nothing if you can't read words
To see the world you need to be brave
Maybe we're all prisoners in Plato's cave
What is the meaning of life?
Why are we here?

Where do we go after we die?
Am I in Plato's cave?
So, if you think you know the world
Is that true or are you blind?
Do you know the games life plays
Or are you also in the cave?

Listening to Meredith sing, thinking about the cave that Parkinson's pulled me out of, I look over at Michael, who wipes a tear from his cheek, and then, with him, I look into the morning light.

Bibliography

Agarwal, Rohan. "Navajos' Art of Deliberate Imperfection." https://michelle alexander.in/blogs/news/navajos.

Berry, Wendell. *Jayber Crow*. Berkeley: Counterpoint, 2001.

Brooks, Gwendolyn. "To Be in Love." http://famouspoetsandpoems.com/poets/ gwendolyn_brooks/poems/4139.

Carel, Havi. *Phenomenology of Illness*. New York: Oxford University Press, 2016.

Cather, Willa. *My Ántonia*. Scotts Valley, CA: CreateSpace, 2018.

Coelho, Paulo. *Veronika Decides to Die*. New York: Harper One, 2006.

Cornwell, Erin York, and Linda J. Waite. "Social Disconnectedness, Perceived Isolation, and Health among Older Adults." *Journal of Health and Social Behavior* 50, no. 1 (2009) 31–48.

Darabont, Frank, dir. *The Shawshank Redemption*. Beverly Hills, CA: Castle Rock Entertainment/Columbia Pictures, 1994.

Day, Dorothy. *The Long Loneliness*. New York: Harper and Row, 1952.

Fox, Michael J. *Always Looking Up: The Adventures of an Incurable Optimist*. New York: Hyperion, 2009.

———. *Lucky Man*. New York: Hachette, 2003.

———. *No Time Like the Future: An Optimist Considers Mortality*. New York: Flatiron, 2020.

Herrick, Robert. "To the Virgins, to Make Much of Time." Poets.org. https:// poets.org/poem/virgins-make-much-time.

Hollingsworth, Heather, and Tammy Webber. "US Tops 500,000 Virus Deaths, Matching the Toll of 3 Wars." https://www.usnews.com/news/health-news /articles/2021-02-22/vaccine-efforts-redoubled-as-us-death-toll-draws-near-500k.

National Academies of Sciences, Engineering, and Medicine. *Social Isolation and Loneliness in Older Adults: Opportunities for the Health Care System*. Washington, DC: The National Academies, 2020.

Rosten, Leo. *Words to Live By: The Real Reason For Being Alive*. Washington, DC: The Sunday Star, 1963.

Rukovets, Olga. "It's a Triple Threat: Loneliness, Parkinson's, and COVID-19." *Neurology Today* 20, no. 22 (November 19, 2020) 8–9. https://journals.lww.com/neurotodayonline/Fulltext/2020/11190/It_s_a_Triple_Threat_Loneliness,_Parkinson_s_and.2.aspx.

Schindler, J. "Perfect Imperfections by Rabbi Judith Schindler." https://temple bethel.org/perfect-imperfections-by-rabbi-judith-schindler/.

Steinbeck, John. *East of Eden*. New York: Penguin, 1952.

———. *Of Mice and Men*. New York: Penguin, 1994.

Tolstoy, Leo. *War and Peace*. New York: Random House, 2007.